THE ULTIMAT_
MACRO DIET
COOKBOOK FOR BEGINNERS

The Complete Macronutrient Guide with 1000 Macro-friendly Recipes for Burning

Stubborn Fat and Gaining Lean Muscle | with 28-day Flexible Macro Diet Meal Plan

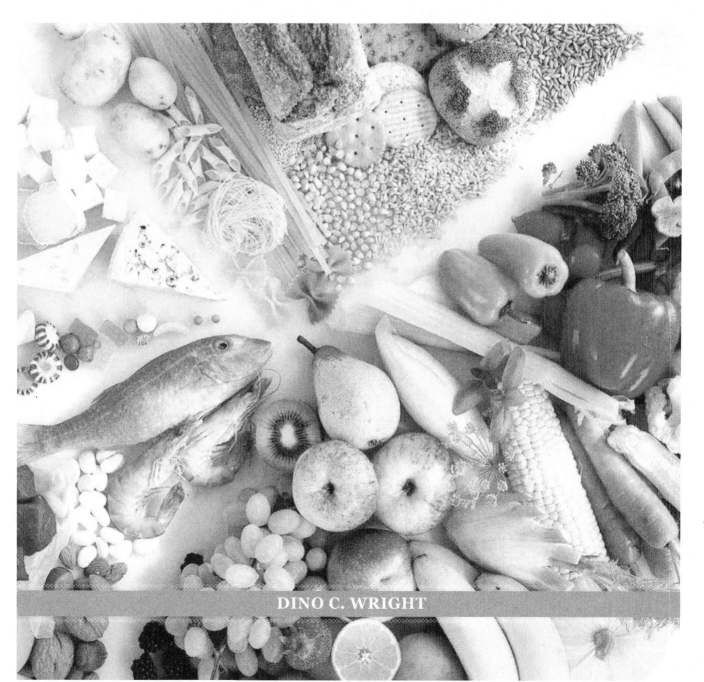

DINO C. WRIGHT

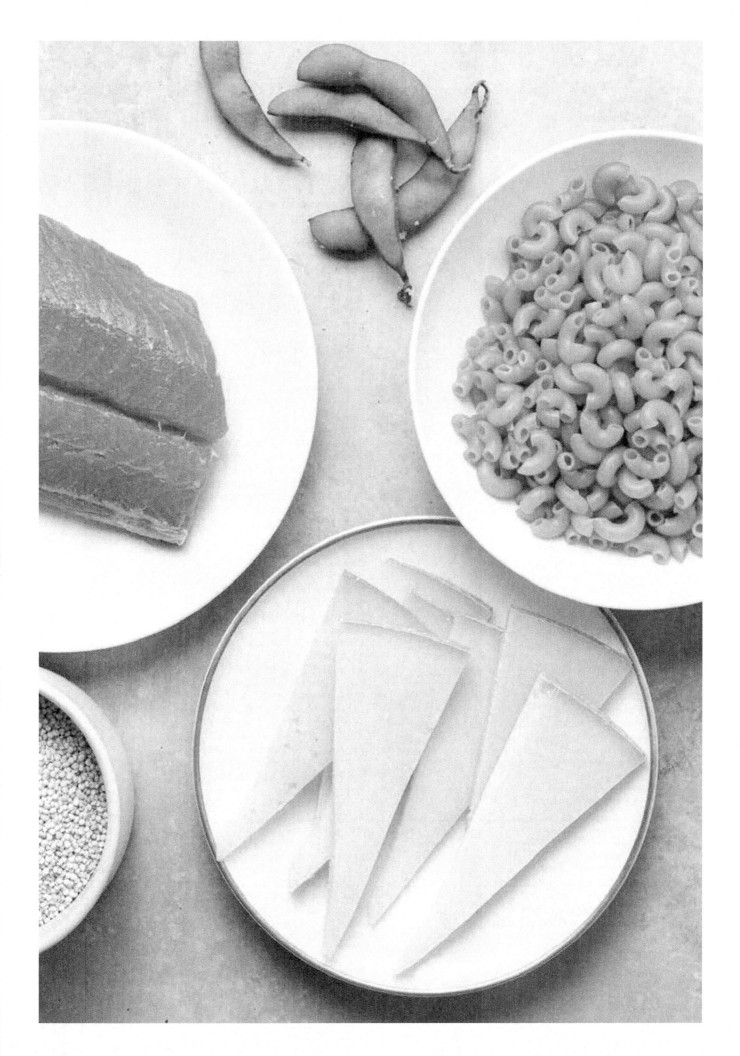

Table of Contents

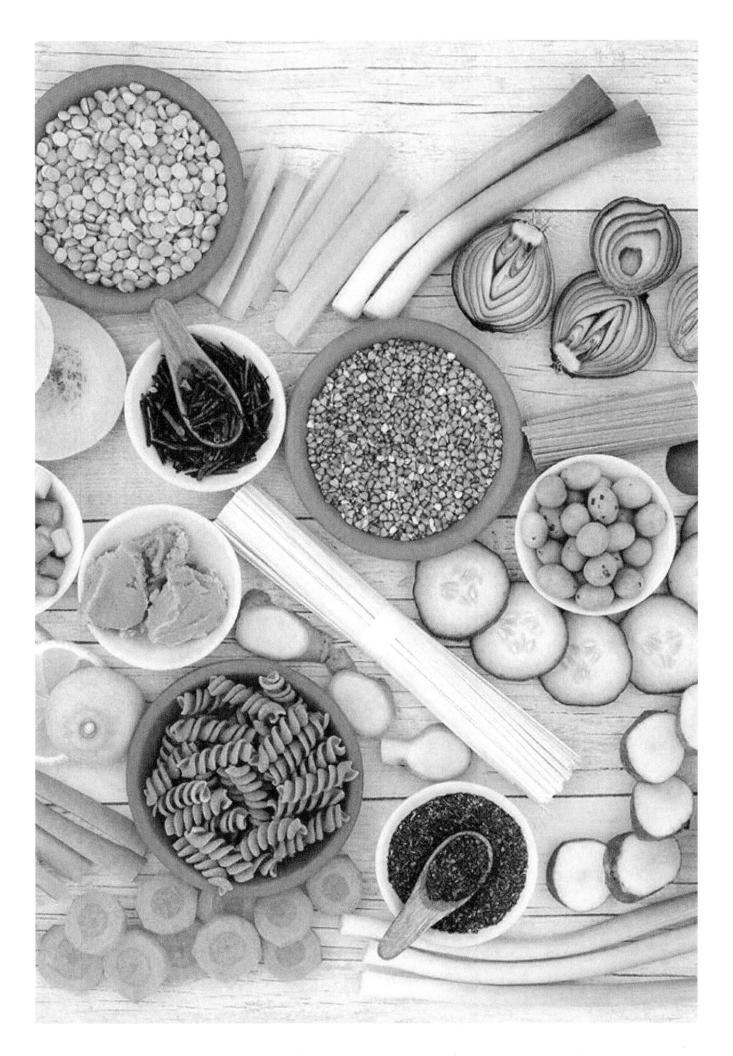

Introduction

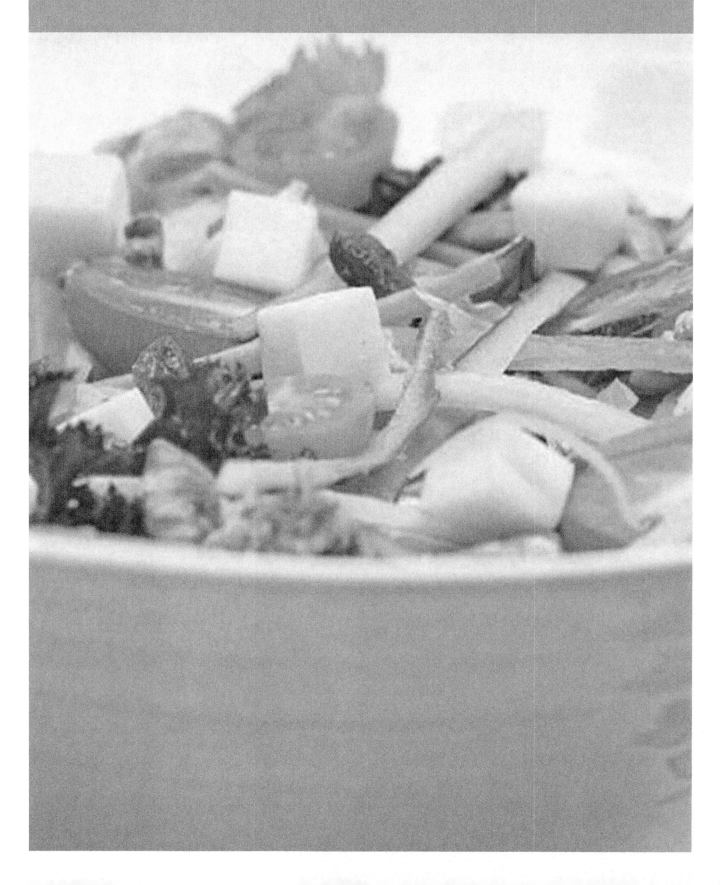

Am I in the right place? You may wonder. It might have been a long journey before finding this cookbook. You could ask yourself many questions about the different books you have used without results. The hard work to find a solution to your problem has been frustrating. It's likely that you are tired and might think this is just any other cookbook.

On the contrary, we have carefully researched and compiled a solution for you. This will be the last cookbook you will ever need. Is it that every time you try a new diet, it fails, or is the fact that your weight loss journey has been compromised, and you now don't know what to do about it? Giving up your favorite dish is not easy. Maybe you are on your body-building journey. Whatever your concerns are, we have a solution for you. You will find a load of information that will walk you through the journey. We have provided all the basic information required, and this book will help you achieve your goal.

Are you worried about the insane rules or the secret body hacks? Not anymore. You can finally say goodbye to the hidden secrets of a new diet. Our book gives results. The stress of spending months relying on a book that promises fast results but leaves you at square one is over. If you are new, we are happy to welcome you. Where there is a will, there is a way. You landing this book means you are willing to make a difference this time. We request that you allow us to show you the way. You shouldn't just read this book and put it back on the shelf. Relax and walk with us. It's a pleasure to bring and walk you through this new diet journey. We want you to understand that we have compiled a guide to help you prepare your diet plan. Following the plan is up to you. We believe you are going to play your part to get results. Before that, let us help you understand the basics of this diet.

Chapter 1
Basics of Macro Diet

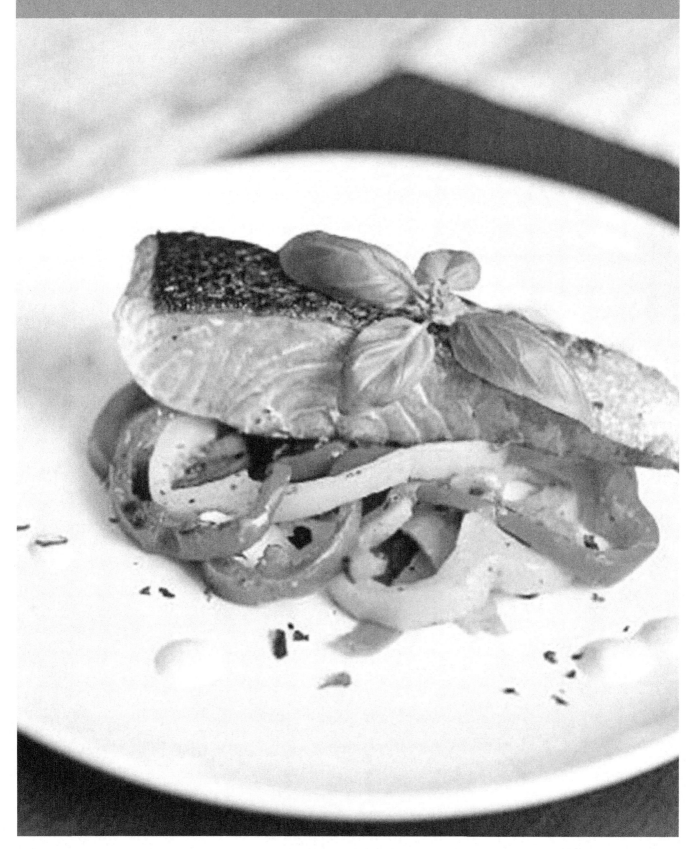

What is a Macro Diet?

To understand a macro diet, you should understand macronutrients. These nutrients are the cornerstones of your diet, macro means large, and therefore macronutrients are nutrients that we require in large quantities that provide us with valuable energy. Carbohydrates, proteins, and fats are macronutrients. It is important to consume these nutrients as they provide energy to the body. They also help us carry out daily activities and maintain body function. A macro diet is a diet that consists of the primary macronutrients, that is, carbohydrates, proteins, and fats. It is a diet plan that focuses on keeping track of nutrients and staying within a certain calorie range. For a successful plan, you must calculate your daily calorie intake and adjust it according to your needs. Your need will depend on the goal you want to achieve. A weight loss journey requires different calories from one who wants to build muscle mass or maintain the right blood sugar levels. This approach may be challenging and time-consuming, but we've made it easier for you.

History of a Macro Diet

Macro comes from the word macrobiotic. Macro and Bio are greek words, "macro" means large or long, and "bio" means life. This diet was first developed by a Greek writer known as Hippocrates. He believed that fresh food and exercise were essential for healthy living. The diet resurfaced again when a famous Prussian physician published a macrobiotics book, "The Art of Prolonging Life" he focused more on natural foods, especially vegetables. Dr. Sagen Ishizuka began the current macro diet. He advocated for simple and natural foods. This is because he realized that when the Japanese ate western foods, disease incidences went up. He aimed to help his parents and other Japanese recover their health. George, a Japanese philosopher, coined the term 'macrobiotic diet.' He believed that eating a healthy and simple diet enabled harmony with nature. He made the macro diet popular around the world. This diet aims to do away with foods containing toxins. George believed this approach could cure cancer, but this is not scientifically proven.

Understand how your Body Works

Your body needs these nutrients to function properly. Once you have served yourself a plate of your plan and started eating, do you know what happens after that? We will help you understand. Digestion begins in the mouth. There are two types of digestion involved, mechanical and chemical. Mechanical digestion happens in the mouth. It involves breaking down the food into smaller pieces through a process known as mastication. After proper digestion in the mouth, the food is swallowed into the esophagus to the stomach, where it undergoes chemical digestion. The organs involved in digesting the food are the oral cavity, stomach, small intestine, liver, gall bladder, and pancreas. The nutrients are further broken down during digestion and used for different functions. These functions include muscle building, cell structure formation, and energy production.

Carbs, short for carbohydrates, are broken down into glucose, protein is broken down into amino acids, and fats into fatty acids and glycerol. All the macronutrients are critical to the body and should be eaten in enough quantities. The recommended amount depends on age, sex, activity level, and other considerations. Athletes and bodybuilders are well suited to this diet. The United States Department of Agriculture Dietary Guideline recommends that adults get at least 130 grams of carbohydrates per day. This amount is enough to provide glucose to your brain. Children and teenagers need more calories, especially fats, to aid brain development; older adults are advised to take more proteins to help preserve muscle mass. Following a strict keto diet or being unable to regulate your insulin level may lead to less glucose in your brain. The great news is that your body will break down fats and proteins to generate energy.

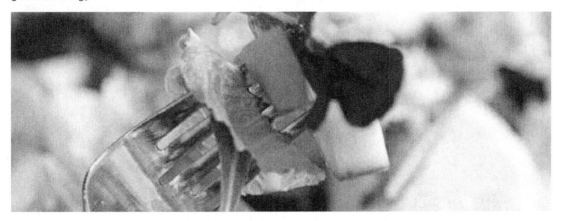

CARBOHYDRATE

A carbohydrate is a biomolecule that consists of carbon, hydrogen, and oxygen. Some carbs, such as uronic acid and fucose, do not conform to this definition. Carbohydrates is a group that consists of starch, sugars, and cellulose. They are found in a variety of natural and processed foods. This means that some carbs are healthier than others. The type of carbs you take is more important than the intake amount. This is an important point to note. There are three primary sources of carbohydrates: sugars, starches, and fiber. Sugars are simple carbohydrates as they contain the most basic form of carbs. These sugars include processed foods, vegetables, milk, and natural fruits. Processed carbs are known as 'bad carbs' some of the foods that fall under this category include sweet and delicious foods such as ice cream, French fries, cookies, cakes, candy, and fruit juice. Starches are referred to as complex carbs consisting of a lot of simple sugars strung together. The body digests starch to produce the energy required for the functioning of your body. Some starches include pasta, cereals, potatoes, corn, and peas. Another type of carbohydrate is fiber- they are also considered complex carbs. Starch and fiber are good carbs. Unlike simple carbs, complex carbs digest slowly. The body does not break down most fibers and, therefore a good choice for weight loss as it leaves you full for longer after eating. Apart from this benefit, fibers will help you prevent constipation and lower blood sugar. Fiber sources consist of whole grains, vegetables, and fruits such as apples, avocados, and berries.

Unlike proteins and fats, carbs are easy to digest and, therefore, the primary energy source in your body. There are two categories of fibers; soluble and insoluble. Soluble fibers dissolve in water while insoluble fibers do not. Due to their soluble nature, these fibers form a gel that helps to improve digestion and reduce blood sugar and cholesterol, reducing the risk of diabetes. Insoluble fibers, on the other hand, attract water to the stool, preventing constipation and reducing the chances of getting diabetes.

WHY DIETARY FIBER?
- It helps with weight loss.
- Normalize bowel movement and helps maintain bowel health.
- Reduces the risk of diabetes.
- Build strong bones. Some soluble fibers such as soybeans and oats help maintain bone density.
- Reduces the chance of breast and colon cancer by controlling estrogen and blood sugar levels.
- You live longer. Dietary fiber reduces the chances of dying from a heart attack.

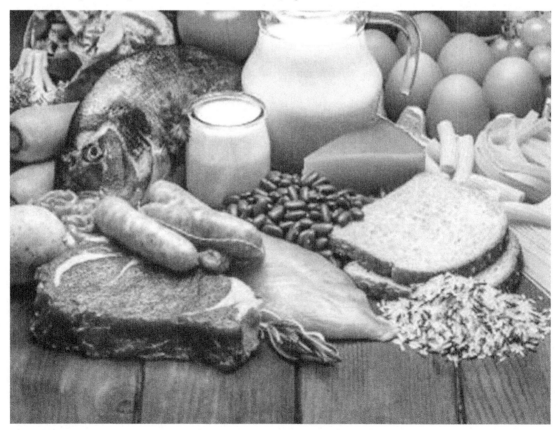

PROTEINS

Proteins are biomolecules that contain a long chain of amino acid residues. They are building blocks of your body, although they can also serve as fuel. In digestion, proteins are broken down into smaller chains through hydrochloric acid and protease action. These actions take place in the stomach. Typically protein digestion begins here. Absorption occurs in the small intestines as the protein is already broken down into amino acids. Proteins have a variety of functions in your body, including DNA replication, catalyzing metabolic reactions, cell and organism structure transportation of molecules, and responding to stimuli. Proteins are essential to your body as they participate in almost all processes within your cells. Most proteins catalyze biochemical reactions and metabolism. They also have both mechanical and structural functions in your body, such as the presence of actin and myosin in muscle and the presence of proteins in the cytoskeleton, which maintains cell shape. To avoid protein-energy malnutrition, ensure your diet is complete. A complete diet has the following essential amino acids; valine, threonine, leucine, histidine, isoleucine, lysine, phenylalanine, tryptophan, and methionine. Your protein is considered incomplete if it lacks any of these amino acids. You may ask yourself what factors to consider to determine your protein intake level. The answer is that it is determined by the overall energy intake, illness or any injury, your body weight and need for amino acids, growth rate, activity level, and the amount of carbs intake.

Other critical considerations include age, pregnancy, and breastfeeding. During childhood, proteins are required in large amounts to aid growth and development. A lactating mum will require a higher intake of proteins to nourish the baby. The United States and Canadian Dietary Reference Intake guidelines recommend that women between the ages of 19-70 consume 46 grams of protein daily to avoid deficiency. Men in the same age bracket, on the other hand, should consume 56 grams per day. These recommendations are for a normal and healthy person. For any concerns, you may consult your dietician.

Plant proteins contribute to a higher percentage of a protein supply. Insects have also been considered protein sources in other parts of the world. The common protein sources include eggs, meat, dairy, soy, fish, cereals, and whole grain. Vegans are not left behind as well. The protein sources include but are not limited to soybeans, kidney beans, mung beans, cashews, lentils, and sesame seeds. Our cookbook provides all the recipes that you may require for this journey. Super easy recipes to cook in the comfort of your home. What un!

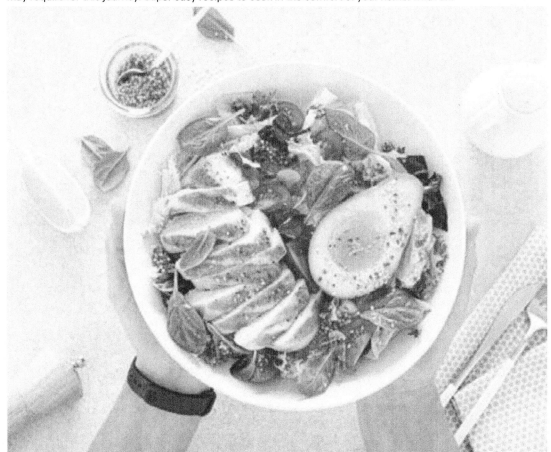

DID YOU KNW TTHERE AARE GOOD FATS?

Fats are sources of fatty acids the body cannot produce. The word fat may sound bad and worrying as fats are associated with body fat (adipose tissue) which most people don't want to hear. Being on your weight loss journey, you do not want the thought of fats in your diet. On the contrary, fat is not all evil. Like other macronutrients, dietary fat is a source of energy. It also helps absorb vitamins A, D, and E in the body. These are fat-soluble vitamins which means they require fats to be absorbed. It's best to understand the difference between dietary and body fat; body fat is the fat you are trying to lose. If you consume more calories than you need, they will be stored in the fat cells causing your body to gain body fat. Dietary fat does not do this. Excess calories from the macronutrients may lead to gaining body fat. This means you shouldn't avoid dietary fats thinking it's the cause of body fat, but rather you should take the right portion of any macronutrient and ensure to take the good fats to avoid health complications. Dietary fats are necessary for the functioning of your body. The main types of fats are:

SATURATED FATS

This is a type of fat where the fatty acid chains have single bonds. Most of these fats come from animal products. Each product has a different amount of saturated fats. The level is higher in processed food, unlike natural foods. Reducing these fats is advisable to limit the risk of health issues such as cardiovascular diseases, diabetes, or death. It is recommended that an average man aged 19-64 years shouldn't have more than 30g of fats in a day; an average woman aged 19-64 years shouldn't have more than 20g of these saturated fats. This fat is found in cheese, bacon, ice cream, butter, coconut and palm oil, biscuits, cakes, sausages, meats, and pastries. These tips will assist you in reducing your intake of saturated fats.

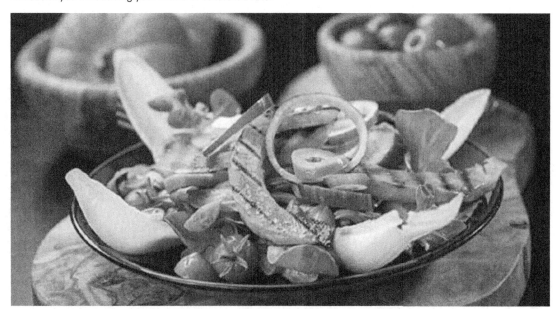

- Take time to compare food labels and pick those lower in saturated fats.
- Limit frying and roasting your foods. You could go for healthier options such as steaming, poaching, and baking.
- Use an oil spray to limit the amount of oil you use during cooking.
- Make your meals at home.
- Remove visible fats on foods such as meat before cooking.
- Go for fish and chicken.
- Cook your food with herbs or spices.
- Consume more vegetables and fruits.

UNSATURATED FAT

Unlike saturated fats are fatty acids where the hydrocarbon molecules have two carbons that share a double or triple bond. They are not saturated with hydrogen atoms. Unsaturated fats are weak in structure and are liquid at room temperature. These fats are mostly found in vegetables and fish. They are a good supply of energy in your body. These fats are classified into two major categories known as monounsaturated and polyunsaturated. Unsaturated fats are healthier than saturated fats as they lower the risk of heart disease. Monounsaturated fats include fats from avocado, pumpkin and sesame seeds, nuts, and olive oils. The other polyunsaturated types include walnuts, fish, soybean, canola oil, and sunflower. Make a choice today. Is it saturated or unsaturated ats?

IS ALCOHOL AA MACRONUTRIENT?

Alcohol is its macronutrient. Since it is not an essential nutrient, it is medically not classified as a macronutrient as the primary three- carbs, proteins, and fats although it has calories like these macros. It has energy contents, but the energy is not stored in the body. That's why it is referred to as a macronutrient of its own. A gram of alcohol contains seven calories, but this calorie is not of any nutritive value. They are known as 'empty calories. In any case, excess alcohol in the body is considered a toxin. If you want to keep track of your calorie intake in a day, you should subtract the number of calories consumed from the alcohol.

WHY DID OTHER DIETS FAIL?

Have you ever wondered why your diet failed or why people complain about not getting results? A big number of the world's population is trying to lose weight in vain, and if successful, they regain it in a few years, sometimes even more weight than before. It is rare for someone to lose weight and maintain it for good. Sometimes it's challenging as you may add weight instead of losing it. The harder you try different diets, the more you add weight. These diets you have tried may have brought about eating disorders and cravings, which isn't a good strategy. You end up not meeting your target and living an unhealthy life. You should grant your body permission to eat what it wants. When you are hindered from doing something, you get tempted to do what you are told not to. That's human nature. This applies to dieting too. If you hinder yourself from eating certain foods, it gives you the urge to eat them, which you do without question. The secret is to permit yourself. It might sound scary, but this is a little secret. In time the desire to eat this food will be less exciting.

WHAT MAKES A MACRO DIFFERENT?

A macro relies on tried and true principles of nutrition. It's not a diet that will promise without giving results. It clears the common rule that there are foods you are not supposed to eat in any diet. Amazingly, in this diet, you will eat what you want as long as you maintain your daily macro target. All you have to do is calculate your daily calorie needs and eat accordingly. To lose weight, you'll have to eat fewer calories than you burn. Macro counting will help you determine this. For example, if you've set a goal for 2000 calories daily, and a gram of proteins contains four calories. Let us say you would like to have 125g of protein. It makes it 500 calories, and you are left with 1500 calories to decide how to use it. Maybe on carbohydrates and fat. With this diet, you have not excluded any of the nutrients. You still have the opportunity to enjoy your favorite food, meet your goal and avoid an unhealthy lifestyle.

AIM TOWARD OPTIMUM FUNCTIONING

The supporting cast of the macro diet is the micronutrients. Unlike macronutrients, they are not a source of energy but are very important for the body's functioning. The body needs micronutrients in small amounts. They provide vitamins and minerals that ensure your body functions optimally. The best way to ensure that you eat a proper amount of these nutrients is to follow the rainbow approach. This means consuming different colored fruits and vegetables. Both macro and micronutrients provide the body with what it requires to stay healthy; hence they work hand in hand. Just like macronutrients, the body doesn't produce micronutrients on its own hence the need for the diet. Vitamins are organic, while minerals are inorganic. When cooked or exposed to acid or air, vitamins can be denatured, making it difficult to ensure you get the nutrients in your diet. Minerals are not affected by the mentioned elements. Therefore, you get all the minerals that your food comes with. Micronutrients are essential for almost all the processes in your body. They act as antioxidants too. A combination of macro and micronutrients is the way to go. Are you coming?

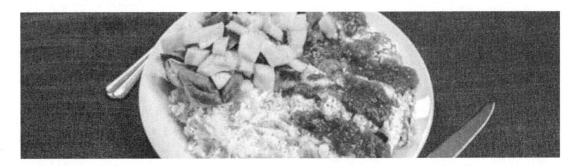

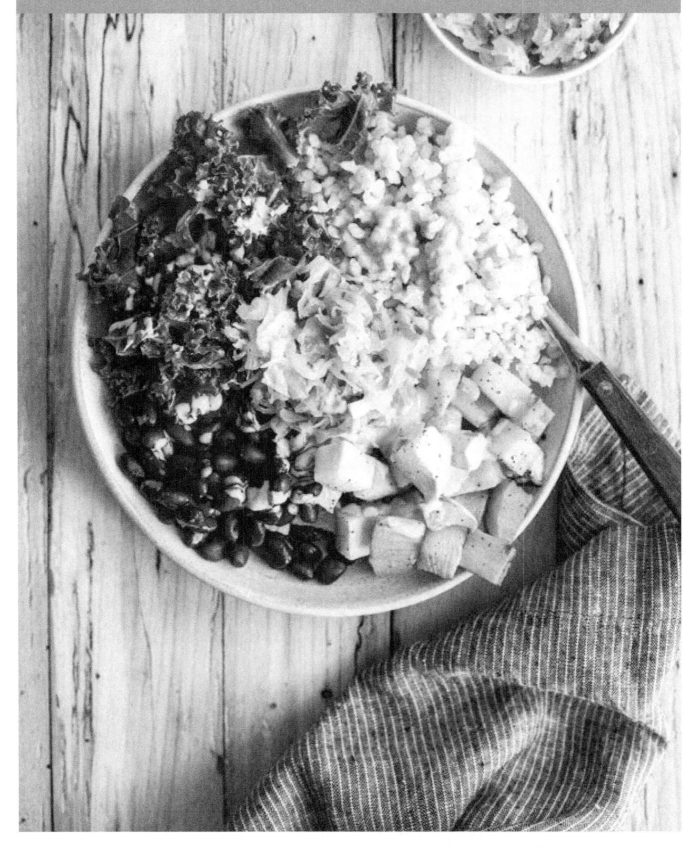

Chater 2
Macro Diet and Body-Building

Have you tried time and again to build muscle mass but every time, it fails? The time spent in the gym and eating a variety of proteins has hit a wall. It must be frustrating. We are here for you. The solution is a macro diet. No matter how hard you try in the gym, lifting weights, the primary factor is proper nutrition. If you invest in a poor diet and spend hours in the gym, your body will not have the necessary raw material to build muscle. Proteins are the foundation of your muscles, so you should be careful with your protein intake amounts if you want to build muscle mass. Inadequate protein is not good for body-building, your body will use up amino in your system to repair any tears, and if you continue going to the gym, you won't gain as expected. Consume enough proteins, then hit the gym for better results. Carbs are also important in muscle building. If you are into body-building, you probably understand how important carbs are, your best friend so far, maybe. Carbs are burnt for immediate fuel and stored in the muscle tissue for later use. This stored glycogen is used during an intense training session. Make carbs your closest friend if you want to start a body-building journey. Fats are also important in this journey. Fats and lean muscle building go hand in hand. They stimulate fat-burning and muscle growth. For better diet results, your macro intake will depend on several factors, they include:

- Body type. It is advisable to determine what your body type is. Are you an endomorph, mesomorph, or ectomorph? Ectomorphs, for example, require a high amount of carbs compared to other body types because of the high metabolism and difficulty in mass gaining. Unlike ectomorphs, mesomorphs are genetically gifted. They have muscles and lower body fat. A moderate carb intake will do for this body type. Endomorphs store more fats; therefore, they need a lower carb intake.
- Gender. Men and females use up macronutrients differently. Men build muscles fast and use glycogen for energy, while women burn fat for fuel. It doesn't mean that men require more carbs than women, but other factors are considered. For example, the gender that exercises more requires more carbs.
- Fitness goals. Whether muscle building or weight loss, keep your goal in mind and eat accrdingly.

Tips to Ensure Success

- Use an app to track your macros. It is advisable to have an app to help you in your journey. Sometimes you may not know how many calories or nutritional information the food you have taken in a day.
- Prepare your meals. You can choose what ingredients to use and how to prepare them. Having readymade food will help you avoid junk or stopping somewhere to eat as you are aware you have to do some eating at your place.
- Try different and new foods. New foods will help you achieve your goal and avoid food boredom.
- Forget preconceived ideas. Some ideas may slow you down. For example, what should or shouldn't be eaten. You can prepare any food anytime you want to have it. If you want to include chicken in your diet, you should do it. A macro diet is not restrictive. Have fun achieving your goal.
- Stay focused. You may often feel pressured to reach your goal and aim for perfection. It's a process, and you will get results.
- Consistency is key, track your macros daily and follow your diet plan to the letter, and your body will reward you.
- Check recipes and menus ahead of time and plan. Going through recipes earlier will make it easy to prepare your meals and avoid skippig them.

Benefits of a Macro Diet

- Psychological benefit, macro diet is not restrictive. It permits you to eat any food as long as you remain within your daily calorie target. It's human nature to go for what they are restricted to. By getting freedom, you escape the trap.
- Physical benefits, you remain in shape and meet your fitness target without restricting yourself. You enjoy the food you love.
- Lifestyle benefit, this diet fits your lifestyle as you do not have to change what you eat. You only have to keep track of your macros.
- A macro diet is an 'everyone' diet. Your goal, body-building, weight loss, or health issues don't matter. This diet will work for you.
- A macro diet is sustainable. It doesn't require any food changes, unlike other diets where it might be challenging to cope for the long term.
- You say goodbye to false hopes. This diet offers results and doesn't take you back to stage one after years of hard work. The result is constant.
- It enables you to be a disciplined individual.

A macro diet is a lifetime solution. We unveil the secret and provide a guide to help you walk through the journey. We aim to show you the way and hand you the light to see you through the tunnel until you are safe on the other side to stand on your own and prepare recipes that suit you without any limitations. That is our joy. Our cookbook will be your all-time book. The hustle is over. You can finally say goodbye to false promises. We understand that you are eager to see what we have prepared for you, so we ain't going to take too much of your time. We wish you all the best and hope you will enjoy the smooth ride to your success. Welcome and have fun!

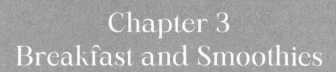

Chapter 3
Breakfast and Smoothies

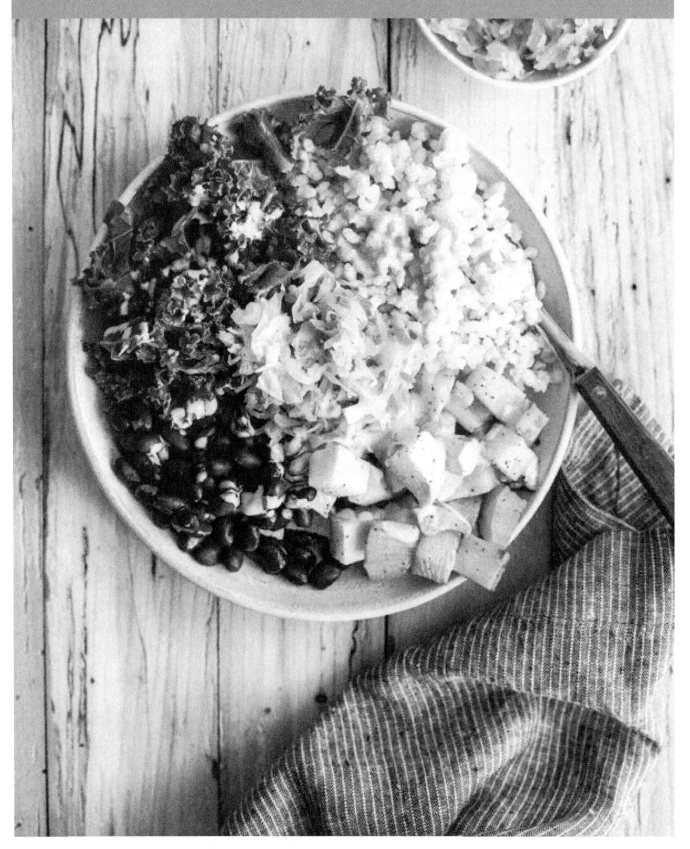

Strawberry Cheesecake Smoothie

Prep time: 5 minutes | Cook time: 5 minutes| Serves 2

- 2 cups (442 grams) frozen strawberries
- 2½ cups (600 milliliters) reduced-fat milk
- 1½ cups (367 grams) nonfat or low-fat plain Greek yogurt
- 2 scoops (68 grams) whey protein powder
- 4 tablespoons (60 grams) low-fat cream cheese

1. In a blender, combine the strawberries, milk, yogurt, whey, and cream cheese. Process on high for 1 to 2 minutes, until smooth.
2. Add more liquid or ice as needed for the desired consistency.

PER SERVING

Calories: 537| Fat: 13g| Protein: 58g| Total Carbs: 48g| Fiber: 5g| Sugar: 37g| Sodium: 408mg

Chocolate and Strawberry Overnight Oats

Prep time: 5 minutes, plus 4 hours to overnight to chill | Cook time: 5 minutes| Serves 2

- 2 cups (162 grams) rolled oats
- 2 cups (475 milliliters) reduced-fat milk
- 1½ cups (367 grams) nonfat or low-fat plain Greek yogurt
- ¼ cup (25 grams) cacao powder
- ¼ cup (60 grams) peanut butter powder
- 3 tablespoons (45 milliliters) maple syrup
- 2 tablespoons (24 grams) chia seeds
- 3 cups (456 grams) sliced fresh strawberries

1. In a large glass bowl, mix the oats, milk, yogurt, cacao powder, peanut butter powder, maple syrup, and chia seeds. Cover and refrigerate for 4 hours or overnight.
2. To serve, top each portion with ½ cup of strawberries.
3. Store for up to five days in the refrigerator to eat throughout the week.

PER SERVING

Calories: 461| Fat: 10g| Protein: 28g| Total Carbs: 67g| Fiber: 14g| Sugar: 27g| Sodium: 183mg

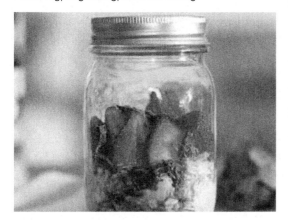

Banana Chia Overnight Oats

Prep time: 5 minutes, plus 4 hours to overnight to chill | Cook time: 5 minutes| Serves 2

- 2 medium ripe bananas (236 grams)
- 2¼ cups (530 milliliters) skim milk
- 2 cups (162 grams) rolled oats
- 1 cup (245 grams) nonfat plain Greek yogurt
- ¼ cup (48 grams) chia seeds
- 1 scoop (34 grams) whey protein powder
- 1 teaspoon (5 milliliters) vanilla extract
- ¼ teaspoon (0.66 gram) ground cinnamon
- 2 tablespoons (31 grams) almond butter

1. In a small bowl, using a fork, mash the bananas well until smooth.
2. Mix in the milk, oats, yogurt, chia seeds, whey, vanilla, and cinnamon. Stir well, cover, and refrigerate for 4 hours or overnight.
3. To serve, top each portion with almond butter.

PER SERVING

Calories: 432| Fat: 11g| Protein: 27g| Total Carbs: 58g| Fiber: 12g| Sugar: 18g| Sodium: 108mg

Protein-Packed French Toast

Prep time: 5 minutes | Cook time: 15 minutes| Serves 4

- 2 large eggs (100 grams)
- 8 large egg whites (267 grams)
- ¼ cup (59 milliliters) unsweetened plain almond milk
- 1 scoop (34 grams) whey protein powder
- ¼ teaspoon (0.66 gram) ground cinnamon
- Dash ground nutmeg (optional)
- Nonstick cooking spray
- 12 whole-grain bread slices (312 grams)
- ¼ cup (30 grams) ground flaxseed
- ¼ cup (64 grams) peanut butter
- ¼ cup (59 milliliters) maple syrup

1. In a large bowl, whisk the eggs, egg whites, almond milk, whey, cinnamon, and nutmeg (if using).
2. Heat a large skillet over medium heat and coat with cooking spray. Dip a piece of bread in the egg mixture, flipping to coat both sides and soak some up.
3. Place the bread in the pan and cook for 2 to 3 minutes on each side, flipping once, until browned. Remove and set aside on a plate. Repeat with the remaining bread, mixing the egg mixture really well each time before you dip the bread to disperse the whey.
4. In a small bowl, thoroughly combine the flaxseed, peanut butter, and maple syrup.
5. Serve the French toast topped with the maple-peanut butter spread.

PER SERVING

Calories: 504| Fat: 18g| Protein: 33g| Total Carbs: 55g| Fiber: 9g| Sugar: 21g| Sodium: 480mg

Egg, Spinach, Scallion, and Feta Burrito

Prep time: 5 minutes | Cook time: 15 minutes| Serves 2

- Nonstick cooking spray
- 4 large eggs (200 grams)
- 4 large egg whites (134 grams)
- 1½ cups (303 grams) cooked brown rice
- 4 cups (120 grams) baby spinach
- 4 scallions (60 grams), both white and green parts, chopped
- 1 tablespoon (9 grams) crumbled feta cheese
- 2 large whole-wheat tortillas (120 grams)
- ½ cup (118 milliliters) salsa

1. Heat a medium skillet over medium-high heat and coat with cooking spray.
2. In a small bowl, scramble the eggs and egg whites. Add them to the skillet and cook for 2 to 4 minutes, stirring regularly, until mostly set.
3. Add the rice, spinach, and scallions and stir for 1 to 2 minutes, until the spinach is wilted. Stir in the feta and mix to combine.
4. Divide the eggs between the tortillas, fold in the sides, and roll up to form a burrito. Cut in half and serve with salsa.

PER SERVING

Calories: 602| Fat: 14g| Protein: 33g| Total Carbs: 80g| Fiber: 9g| Sugar: 7g| Sodium: 1047mg

Sweet Potato and Turkey Hash with Eggs

Prep time: 5 minutes | Cook time: 15 minutes| Serves 4

- 1 pound (454 grams) lean ground turkey
- Nonstick cooking spray
- 2 sweet potatoes (260 grams), shredded
- ¼ teaspoon (1.5 grams) salt
- ¼ teaspoon (0.58 gram) freshly ground black pepper
- 8 large eggs (400 grams)
- ¼ cup (15 grams) chopped parsley

1. In a large skillet over medium heat, cook the turkey for about 5 minutes, breaking up, until cooked through. If not using a nonstick skillet, add a little water to the skillet to prevent sticking. Remove from the pan and set aside.
2. Coat the skillet with cooking spray and return to medium heat. Add the sweet potatoes and cook, flipping gently with a spatula every couple of minutes, for about 10 minutes, until browned and crispy. Add the salt and pepper.
3. Mix the turkey back into the skillet and gently stir. Transfer to serving plates or containers.
4. Coat the skillet with cooking spray and return to medium heat. Crack the eggs into the pan in batches and cook for 2 to 3 minutes, until set. Flip and cook for another 1 to 3 minutes, until preferred doneness.

5. Serve each portion of hash topped with eggs and garnished with parsley.

PER SERVING

Calories: 454| Fat: 24g| Protein: 45g| Total Carbs: 15g| Fiber: 2g| Sugar: 4g| Sodium: 411mg

Hard-Boiled Egg, Roasted Potato, and Spinach Breakfast Bowl

Prep time: 15 minutes | Cook time: 15 minutes| Serves 4

- 1 pound (453 grams) small new potatoes
- Nonstick cooking spray
- 8 large hard-boiled eggs (400 grams), peeled and chopped
- 8 hard-boiled egg whites (235 grams), peeled and chopped
- Salt
- Freshly ground black pepper
- 8 cups (240 grams) chopped spinach
- 2 cups (370 grams) cooked quinoa
- 4 scallions (60 grams), both white and green parts, chopped
- ½ cup (118 milliliters) parsley, garlic, and sunflower seed sauce

1. Preheat the oven to broil on high.
2. Place the potatoes in a large microwave-safe bowl that has a lid. Cover loosely with the lid and cook for 5 to 7 minutes, until the potatoes are tender.
3. Transfer the potatoes to a baking sheet and, using the bottom of a glass, smash the potatoes gently and coat lightly with cooking spray. Transfer to the oven and broil for 5 to 8 minutes, until browned.
4. Divide the potatoes between bowls and top each with 2 hard-boiled eggs and 2 hard-boiled egg whites. Season with salt and pepper. Add 2 cups of chopped spinach and ½ cup of quinoa to each bowl. Divide the scallions over the top of each portion and drizzle with the sauce.

PER SERVING

Calories: 450| Fat: 20g| Protein: 29g| Total Carbs: 39g| Fiber: 7g| Sugar: 4g| Sodium: 641mg

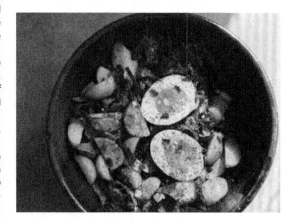

Shakshuka with Spinach

Prep time: 5 minutes | Cook time: 20 minutes | Serves 4

- 1 tablespoon (15 milliliters) extra-virgin olive oil
- 1 small yellow onion (70 grams), chopped
- 1 medium red bell pepper (119 grams), seeded and chopped
- 3 garlic cloves (9 grams), minced
- 2 (15-ounce) cans (847 grams) diced tomatoes
- 2 cups (220 grams) grated carrots
- 1½ teaspoons (3.4 grams) paprika
- 1 teaspoon (2 grams) ground cumin
- ½ teaspoon (3 grams) salt
- 4 cups (120 grams) chopped spinach
- 8 large eggs (400 grams)
- 8 large egg whites (267 grams)
- ½ cup (30 grams) chopped parsley

1. In a large skillet, heat the oil over medium heat. Cook the onion and bell pepper for about 5 minutes, stirring occasionally, until softened. Add the garlic and sauté for 30 seconds, until fragrant.
2. Add the tomatoes and carrots and mix well. Stir in the paprika, cumin, and salt. Bring to a simmer and cook for about 5 minutes, until slightly thickened.
3. Stir in the spinach. Then, using a large spoon, make 8 wells in the mixture, evenly spaced throughout the skillet. Crack an egg into each well and pour the egg whites on top of the eggs. Cover and cook for 5 to 8 minutes, until cooked to your desired doneness.
4. Garnish with chopped parsley and serve.

PER SERVING

Calories: 327| Fat: 15g| Protein: 24g| Total Carbs: 24g| Fiber: 7g| Sugar: 12g| Sodium: 949mg

Cinnamon Applesauce Oatmeal

Prep time: 10 minutes | Cook time: 6 minutes | Serves 4

- 6 large egg whites
- ½ cup oatmeal
- 1 tablespoon unsweetened applesauce
- 1 teaspoon cinnamon
- 1 packet stevia
- ¼ teaspoon baking soda
- 1 teaspoon olive oil
- 1 medium apple, diced

1. Heat a medium nonstick pan over medium heat for 5 minutes.
2. Combine all ingredients except oil and apple in a blender, blending until mixed well.
3. Lightly oil the pan, coating all surfaces.
4. Slowly pour 1/4 of batter into the pan.
5. When mixture starts to bubble, top with 1/4 of apples and flip.
6. Cook 1 more minute, then serve immediately.

PER SERVING (1 PANCAKE)

Calories: 386 | Fat: 8 g | Protein: 27 g | Sodium: 646 mg | Fiber: 8 g | Carbohydrates: 55 g | Sugar: 20 g

Egg and Applesauce Banana Muffins

Prep time: 15 minutes | Cook time: 30 minutes | Serves 12

- 1 ¼ cups whole-wheat flour
- ³/4 teaspoon baking soda
- ½ teaspoon salt
- 2 tablespoons unsalted butter, softened
- ¼ cup brown sugar (or stevia alternative)
- 2 large egg whites
- 3 ripe medium bananas
- ¼ cup pure maple syrup
- 2 tablespoons unsweetened applesauce
- ½ teaspoon vanilla extract
- ⅓ cup crushed pecans

1. Preheat oven to 325°F (163°C).
2. Line a 12-cup muffin tin with baking liners.
3. Combine flour, baking soda, and salt in a large bowl and mix well.
4. In a separate large bowl, mix butter and brown sugar until smooth.
5. Add egg whites, bananas, maple syrup, applesauce, and vanilla and mix by hand or with an electric mixer until well blended.
6. Gently stir in flour mixture until combined and then evenly divide into lined muffin cups.
7. Sprinkle muffin tops with pecans and bake 30–35 minutes, until a toothpick inserted into the center comes out clean.

PER SERVING (1 MUFFIN)

Calories: 143 | Fat: 5 g | Protein: 3 g | Sodium: 191 mg | Fiber: 2.5 g | Carbohydrates: 25 g | Sugar: 7 g

Vanilla Whipped Protein Bowl

Prep time: 5 minutes | Cook time: 0 minute | Serves 1

- ½ cup fat-free Greek yogurt
- 1 scoop vanilla whey protein
- ¼ cup water
- 1 cup frozen mixed berries
- ½ cup fat-free whipped cream

1. Combine yogurt, protein, and water in a small bowl, whisking until blended.
2. Let bowl sit in freezer 5 minutes to thicken.
3. Remove from freezer, top with berries and whipped cream, and serve.

PER SERVING

Calories: 333 | Fat: 8 g | Protein: 38 g | Sodium: 86 mg | Fiber: 3.5 g | Carbohydrates: 30 g | Sugar: 22 g

Egg and Tortilla Spinach Wrap

Prep time: 10 minutes | Cook time: 5 minutes | Serves 1

- Cooking spray
- 3 large egg whites
- 1 cup chopped baby spinach
- ¼ cup feta cheese
- 2 tablespoons sun-dried tomatoes, chopped
- 1 medium whole-wheat tortilla

1. Heat a medium skillet over medium heat and coat lightly with cooking spray.
2. Scramble egg whites and spinach until fully cooked.
3. Add feta cheese and mix well.
4. Spread tomatoes in tortilla, add egg mixture, roll, and serve.

PER SERVING

Calories: 175 | Fat: 8.5 g | Protein: 18 g | Sodium: 549 mg | Fiber: 1.5 g | Carbohydrates: 7 g | Sugar: 5 g

Mango Green Smoothie

Prep time: 5 minutes | Cook time: 5 minutes | Serves 4

- 2 bananas, preferably frozen, peeled and sliced
- 3 cups fresh baby spinach
- 1 1/2 cups diced fresh mango (about 2 mangos)
- 1/4 cup shelled raw hemp seeds
- 3 1/4 cups 2% milk
- 2 cups ice cubes

1. Into a blender, add banana slices, spinach, mango, hemp seeds, milk, and ice.
2. Blend until smooth, pour into 4 glasses, and serve.

PER SERVING

Calories: 271 | protein: 12g | carbs: 37g | fat: 9g

Green Smoothie Bowl with Berries

Prep time: 8 minutes | Cook time: 5 minutes | Serves 2

- 2 medium fresh or frozen bananas (236 grams)
- 2 cups (42 grams) chopped kale
- 1½ cups (350 milliliters) plain unsweetened almond milk
- 1½ cups (228 grams) fresh or frozen strawberries
- ½ avocado (75 grams), peeled and pitted
- ½ cup (40 grams) rolled or instant oats
- ¼ cup (35 grams) sunflower seeds
- ¼ cup (31 grams) fresh berries of choice

1. In a blender, combine the bananas, kale, almond milk, strawberries, avocado, oats, and whey. Process until smooth and pour into two bowls.
2. Top each bowl with the sunflower seeds and berries to serve.

PER SERVING

Calories: 561 | Fat: 20g | Protein: 36g | Total Carbs: 66g | Fiber: 14g | Sugar: 27g | Sodium: 248mg

Mass Building Sweet Potato Pancakes

Prep time: 5 minutes | Cook time: 15 minutes | Serves 4

- 1 medium sized sweet potato
- 1 egg
- 4 egg whites
- 8oz fat-free Greek yogurt
- 1/2 cup of oats
- 1 tsp cinnamon
- 1 tsp vanilla extract
- 1 tsp of honey
- Handful of diced strawberries
- Handful of blueberries

1. Rinse sweet potato under cold water for a couple of seconds and then pierce it with a fork several times and place it in the microwave until soft (about 8 minutes).
2. After let it cool down before removing all skin with a knife.
3. Put the oats into a blender and blend until they are a fine powder, then place into a bowl.
4. Place the sweet potato in the blender and blend until smooth, and then mix with the powdered oats.
5. Add the egg, egg whites, vanilla, cinnamon, honey and yogurt and stir well. This is now your pancake batter.
6. Spray a pan with cooking spray and place over medium heat. Pour roughly a quarter of the batter into the pan and cook for 1-2 minutes. Flip the pancake and cook for another 30 seconds
7. Once done, remove your tasty pancake and top with the berries.
8. Use the same method for the rest of your batter.

PER SERVING

Calories: 451 | protein: 38g Carbs: 74g | fat: 9g

Peanut Butter Banana Smoothie

Prep time: 5 minutes | Cook time: 5 minutes | Serves 2

- 1 medium banana (118 grams)
- 1½ cups (350 milliliters) skim milk
- ¾ cup (184 grams) nonfat or low-fat plain Greek yogurt
- 1 cup ice
- 2 scoops (68 grams) whey protein powder
- 2 tablespoons (32 grams) peanut butter
- 2 tablespoons (15 grams) ground flaxseed
- 1 tablespoon (15 milliliters) maple syrup

1. In a blender, combine the banana, milk, yogurt, ice, whey, peanut butter, flaxseed, and maple syrup. Process on high for 1 to 2 minutes, until smooth.
2. Add more liquid or ice as needed for the desired consistency.

PER SERVING

Calories: 467 | Fat: 13g | Protein: 48g | Total Carbs: 42g | Fiber: 4g | Sugar: 32g | Sodium: 214mg

Brawny Breakfast Burrito

Prep time: 5 minutes | Cook time: 10 minutes| Serves 4

- 2 eggs
- 1/2 cup of low fat milk
- 1/4 cup of black beans
- 4oz of low fat cheese
- Handful of chopped red peppers
- 1 tsp of chopped coriander
- 1 tbsp of salsa
- ½ tsp of cumin

1. Add the milk, eggs and cumin to a bowl and whisk together.
2. Spray pan with cooking spray and place over medium heat. Add the mixture to the pan. After roughly 2 – 3 minutes, add the low fat cheese, chopped red peppers and black beans to the omelette.
3. Once added fold the omelette in half and let it cook through (1-2 minutes).
4. Remove from pan and serve with the salsa and coriander.

PER SERVING

Calories: 302 | protein: 25g Carbs: 19g|fat: 16g

Super Scrambled Turkey Bacon Eggs On Toast

Prep time: 5 minutes | Cook time: 5 minutes| Serves 4

- 6 egg whites
- 3 slices of turkey bacon
- 2 slices of Ezekiel or wholemeal bread
- Handful of chopped onion
- Handful of chopped yellow peppers
- Handful of chopped white mushrooms
- 1 tsp of garlic powder
- 1 tsp of dried parsley
- 1 tsp of olive oil

1. Spray pan with cooking spray and place over medium/high heat. Add the chopped onions, chopped yellow peppers and white mushrooms and cook until soft.
2. In a different pan, cook the turkey bacon.
3. Add the egg whites and garlic powder to the pan with the veggies and 1tsp of olive oil and scramble until the eggs become firm.
4. Toast the Ezekiel bread.
5. Break up the turkey bacon and add to the scrambled eggs
6. Plate up and serve scrambled eggs and turkey bacon on bread, sprinkled with the fresh parsley.
7. Add salt and pepper as required.

PER SERVING

Calories: 299 | protein: 22g Carbs: 35g|fat: 8g

Banana and Almond Muscle Oatmeal

Prep time: 5 minutes | Cook time: 8 minutes| Serves 4

- 1/2 cup of rolled oats
- 1 cup of low fat milk
- 1 scoop of whey protein (vanilla or chocolate)
- Handful of chopped almonds
- 1 tsp of organic peanut butter
- 1 diced banana

1. Throw the oats and low fat milk into a large bowl, stir and place in the microwave for two minutes.
2. Add the diced banana, peanut butter, whey protein and chopped almonds to the oats and mix in.

PER SERVING

Calories: 523 | protein: 32gCarbs: 16g|fat: 15g

Egg and Chocolate French Toast

Prep time: 10 minutes | Cook time: 3 minutes | Serves 1

- Cooking spray
- 3 large egg whites
- ½ scoop chocolate protein powder
- 2 slices whole-grain bread
- 1 packet stevia
- 1 teaspoon cinnamon
- ½ cup sugar-free maple syrup

1. Heat a medium skillet over medium-high heat and coat lightly with cooking spray.
2. Whisk together egg whites and protein in a large bowl.
3. Dip bread into egg and protein mixture, coating both sides.
4. 4. Add slices to skillet, cooking 2–3 minutes per side or until golden brown.
5. 5. Remove from skillet; top with stevia, cinnamon, and syrup. Serve immediately.

PER SERVING

Calories: 295 | Fat: 2 g | Protein: 29 g | Sodium: 689 mg | Fiber: 3 g | Carbohydrates: 46 g | Sugar: 7 g

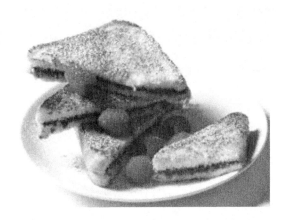

Blueberry-Coconut Pancake Batter Smoothie

Prep time: 5 minutes | Cook time: 5 minutes| Serves 1

- 1/2 cup coconut water
- 1 cup low-fat buttermilk
- 1/4 cup 2% cottage cheese
- 1/4 cup 2% Greek yogurt
- 1 tablespoon coconut flour
- 2 tablespoons honey or date paste
- 1 tablespoon shredded unsweetened coconut
- 1/2 teaspoon baking soda
- 1/4 cup fresh blueberries, plus more for garnish

1. Into a blender, add coconut water, buttermilk, cottage cheese, yogurt, coconut flour, honey, coconut, and baking soda. Blend until smooth.
2. Add blueberries and pulse a few times just until slightly broken up.
3. Pour the pancake smoothie into a glass and garnish with a small handful of blueberries. Serve.

PER SERVING

Calories:431 | protein: 24g| carbs: 67g|fat: 9g

Apple Pie Smoothie

Prep time: 5 minutes | Cook time: 5 minutes| Serves 2

- 2 large apples (446 grams), cored
- 2 cups (475 milliliters) reduced-fat milk
- 1 cup (245 grams) nonfat or low-fat plain Greek yogurt
- 1 cup (30 grams) baby spinach, packed
- 1 cup ice
- 2 scoops (68 grams) whey protein powder
- ¼ cup (30 grams) ground flaxseed
- 2 pitted dates (48 grams)
- 2 teaspoons (10 milliliters) avocado oil or extra-virgin olive oil
- ½ teaspoon (1.32 grams) ground cinnamon

1. In a blender, combine the apples, milk, yogurt, spinach, ice, whey, flaxseed, dates, oil, and cinnamon. Process on high for 1 to 2 minutes, until smooth.
2. Add more liquid or ice as needed for the desired consistency.

PER SERVING

Calories: 638| Fat: 17g| Protein: 52g| Total Carbs: 74g| Fiber: 12g| Sugar: 60g| Sodium: 272mg

Protein Powered Pancakes

Prep time: 5 minutes | Cook time: 10 minutes| Serves 2 (Makes about 5 pancakes)

- 6 egg whites
- 1/2 cup of rolled oats
- 1 tsp flaxseed oil
- 1 tsp of cinnamon
- 1 tsp of stevia

1. Put the oats and all the other ingredients into a blender and blend. This is now your pancake batter.
2. Spray pan with cooking spray and place over medium heat.
3. Pour roughly 1/5 of the pancake batter into the pan and cook for 1-2 minutes. Flip the pancake and cook for another 30 seconds.
4. Once done, remove your tasty pancake.
5. Use the same method for the rest of your batter.

PER SERVING

Calories: 337 | protein: 27g,Carbs: 33g|fat: 9g

Turkey Muscle Omelette

Prep time: 5 minutes | Cook time: 15 minutes| Serves 2

- 10oz of chopped or minced turkey
- 3 eggs
- Handful of baby spinach
- Handful of kale
- 1 tbsp of olive oil
- 1/4 cup of low fat cheese

1. Crack the eggs into a bowl and whisk.
2. Grab a pan and heat half the oil on a medium heat, then add the turkey, kale and cheese and cook for 5-6 minutes.
3. In a different pan, heat the rest of the olive oil and then add the eggs and cook for around 4 minutes.
4. Add the turkey mix into the pan with the eggs and sprinkle some baby spinach on top, then fold the omelette in half.
5. Cook for another 2-3 minutes.
6. Plate up and serve.

PER SERVING

Calories: 358 | protein: 26g|carbs: 5g|fat: 21g

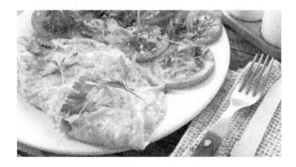

Cottage Cheese Berry Bowl

Prep time: 5 minutes | Cook time: 5 minutes| Serves 4

- 4 cups (904 grams) reduced-fat cottage cheese
- 6 cups (738 grams) raspberries, blueberries, or blackberries
- 4 tablespoons (28 grams) slivered or chopped almonds or walnuts
- 6 tablespoons (30 grams) unsweetened shredded coconut
- 6 tablespoons (90 milliliters) maple syrup

1. In a food processor, combine the cottage cheese and berries and pulse until mixed well.
2. Transfer to bowls to serve and top with the nuts, coconut, and a drizzling of maple syrup.

PER SERVING

Calories: 888| Fat: 30g| Protein: 56g| Total Carbs: 112g| Fiber: 28g| Sugar: 72g| Sodium 1408mg

Aesthetic Asparagus Frittata

Prep time: 5 minutes | Cook time: 20 minutes| Serves 3

- 2 cups of chopped asparagus
- ½ broccoli (florets only)
- 8 eggs
- Handful of chopped parsley
- 1 tsp of chives
- 1 tbsp of olive oil
- 1 cup of low fat milk
- Salt and pepper

1. Crack the eggs into a bowl, add the milk and some salt and pepper and whisk.
2. Get a covered skillet and steam the broccoli over a medium heat for 4-5 minutes. Set to one side.
3. Next, in the same skillet, heat the oil. Add the chopped asparagus, chopped parsley and chives into the skillet and cook for around 2-3 minutes on a medium heat.
4. Add the egg mixture, along with the broccoli into the skillet and cover the skillet evenly.
5. Cook for around 3-4 minutes or until the eggs are set right through
6. Take the skillet and place under the grill for around 2 minutes or until the top is golden (optional).
7. Plate up and serve.

PER SERVING

Calories: 349 | protein: 23g,Carbs: 8g|fat: 25g

Avocado-Mint Protein Smoothie

Prep time: 5 minutes | Cook time: 5 minutes| Serves 1

- 1 cup unsweetened almond milk
- 4 fresh mint leaves
- 1 banana, peeled and sliced
- 1/2 medium avocado, peeled and pitted
- 3 whole dates (2.5 ounces), pitted
- 1 tablespoon dark chocolate chips
- 1 scoop vanilla protein powder

1. Into a blender, add almond milk, mint, banana, avocado, dates, chocolate chips, and protein powder.
2. Blend ingredients until smooth. Pour smoothie into a glass and serve.

PER SERVING

Calories: 664| protein: 29g| carbs: 103g|fat: 22g

Crispy Rice Skillet

Prep time 10 minutes | Cook time 15 minutes| Serves 2

- 2 cups liquid egg whites
- $\frac{1}{2}$ tsp ground ginger
- $\frac{1}{8}$ tsp red pepper flakes
- 1 tsp liquid aminos
- 1 cup frozen peas
- 2 tbsp finely chopped scallions (green parts only)
- 1 tsp minced garlic
- 1 cup cooked basmati rice

1. Preheat the broiler to low. In a large bowl, make the egg mixture by whisking together the egg whites, ginger, red pepper flakes, and liquid aminos. Add the peas to the bowl, and stir well to combine. Set aside.
2. Spray a medium cast iron skillet with non-stick cooking spray and preheat over medium heat. Add the scallions and garlic, and cook for 2 to 3 minutes until soft and fragrant.
3. Increase the heat to medium-high, add the rice to the skillet, and use a wooden spoon to spread it into a thin, even layer. Toast for 1 to 2 minutes. Use the wooden spoon to press the rice into the skillet and toast for an additional 1 to 2 minutes, or until the rice is brown and crispy.
4. Reduce the heat to low. Pour the egg mixture evenly over the toasted rice. Cook for 4 to 5 minutes, then transfer the skillet to the oven. Broil for 2 to 3 minutes, or until the egg whites are set. Serve hot.

PER SERVING

Calories: 278|fat:0.5g|carbs: 321g| protein: 33.9g

Steamed Squash Egg Custard

Prep time 10 minutes | Cook time 45 minutes| Serves 4

- 4 medium acorn squash
- 4 cups liquid egg whites
- 4 tbsp coconut milk
- 1 tbsp powdered stevia
- 1 tsp ground cinnamon
- 1 tsp pumpkin pie spice

1. Using a sharp knife, carefully cut a large hole around the stem of each squash. Remove the stems and reserve for later, and use a spoon to scoop out and discard the seeds.
2. Fill the bottom of a large pot with 1 inch (2.5cm) water. Place a steaming tray in the pot, cover, and heat the water on medium-low until just simmering.
3. In a large bowl, combine the egg whites, coconut milk, stevia, cinnamon, and pumpkin pie spice. Mix well.
4. Pour equal amounts of the egg mixture into each squash. Place the stems back on the squash and place them upright in the pot. Cover, and steam for 45 minutes.
5. Using tongs, carefully remove the squash from the pot and transfer to a plate. Allow to cool slightly before serving.

PER SERVING

Calories:268 |fat:0.3g|carbs: 33.1g| protein: 32.7g

Breakfast Hash

Prep time 10 minutes | Cook time 25 minutes| Serves 4

- 1 medium white onion, diced
- 1lb (450g) ground turkey breast
- 1 tsp ground cumin
- 1 tsp red pepper flakes
- 1 tsp paprika
- 1 tsp salt
- 2 medium sweet potatoes, peeled and cut into $\frac{1}{2}$-inch (1.25cm) cubes
- 2 cups fresh baby spinach
- 4 medium eggs

1. Preheat the broiler to low. Spray a medium cast iron skillet with coconut oil cooking spray and place over medium heat.
2. Add the onion to the skillet. Cook until soft and translucent, stirring frequently. Add the turkey breast, cumin, red pepper flakes, paprika, and salt. Stir well to combine, using a wooden spoon to break up the ground turkey. Cook for 6 to 8 minutes, stirring frequently, until the turkey is browned. Transfer to a large bowl and set aside.
3. Add the sweet potatoes to the skillet and cook for 8 to 10 minutes, or until soft. Add the spinach and cook for an additional 1 to 2 minutes, or until wilted. Add the turkey and onions back to the skillet. Mix well.
4. Make 4 divots in the hash and carefully crack an egg into each divot. Place the skillet in the oven and broil for 5 to 7 minutes, or until the eggs are set and the hash is lightly browned. Serve hot.

PER SERVING

Calories: 292|fat:6.6g|carbs: 23g| protein: 35g

Low-Carb Pancake

Prep time 10 minutes | Cook time 15 minutes| Serves 1

- 1 cup liquid egg whites
- $\frac{1}{3}$ cup unsweetened almond milk
- $\frac{1}{2}$ tsp vanilla extract
- 2 tbsp coconut flour
- $\frac{1}{8}$ cup almond flour
- $\frac{1}{2}$ tsp baking powder
- $\frac{1}{4}$ tsp ground cinnamon
- $\frac{1}{2}$ tsp powdered stevia
- 2 tbsp no-calorie pancake syrup (optional)

1. In a medium bowl, combine the egg whites, almond milk, and vanilla extract. Stir well. In a separate medium bowl, combine the coconut flour, almond flour, baking powder, cinnamon, and stevia. Mix well.
2. Make the batter by adding the wet ingredients to the dry ingredients. Mix well, and allow the batter to thicken for 10 minutes.
3. Spray a medium skillet with non-stick cooking spray and preheat over medium-high heat. Pour the batter into the hot pan, and cook until the edges are set and bubbles appear on the surface. Flip, and cook for 1 additional minute. Transfer the cooked pancake to a plate.
4. Drizzle with the syrup (if using). Serve warm.

PER SERVING

Calories:275 |fat:9.8g|carbs: 13.5g| protein: 33.5g

Pumped-Up Protein Pancake

Prep time 10 minutes | Cook time 15 minutes| Serves 1

- 1 cup liquid egg whites
- $\frac{1}{2}$ cup old-fashioned oats
- 1 tbsp coconut flour
- $\frac{1}{2}$ tsp ground cinnamon
- $\frac{1}{2}$ tsp baking powder
- 2 tbsp no-calorie pancake syrup (optional)

1. In a medium bowl, combine the egg whites, oats, coconut flour, cinnamon, and baking powder. Mix well, and allow to thicken for 5 to 10 minutes.
2. Spray a medium skillet with non-stick cooking spray and preheat over medium heat.
3. Add the batter to the hot pan, cover, and cook for 10 to 12 minutes. Transfer the cooked pancake to a plate.
4. Drizzle with the syrup (if using). Serve warm.

PER SERVING

Calories:300 |fat:3.7g|carbs: 36g| protein: 30g

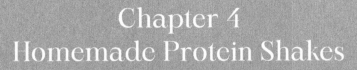

Chapter 4
Homemade Protein Shakes

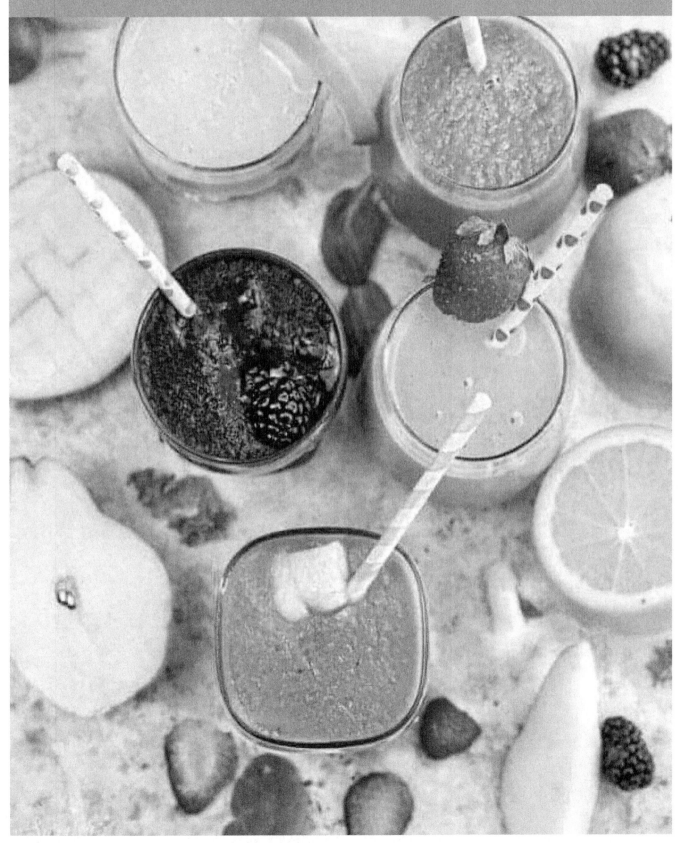

Green and Mean

Prep time: 5 minutes | Cook time: 5 minutes| Serves 1

- 3 stalks of celery
- 3 bunches of kale
- ½ cup of sliced pineapple
- ½ apple, chopped
- A handful of spinach
- 1 tbsp of coconut oil
- 1 scoop of vanilla protein powder

1. Place all the ingredients together in the blender and process until the desired consistency is achieved.
2. Pour contents of the blender into a tall glass. Serve immediately and enjoy!

PER SERVING

Calories: 497 | protein: 28g|carbs: 62g|fat: 17g

Chocolate Peanut Delight

Prep time: 5 minutes | Cook time: 5 minutes| Serves 1

- 1 scoop of chocolate whey protein powder
- 1 cup of low-fat Greek yogurt
- 1 whole banana
- 2 tbsp of peanut butter
- 1 cup of ice

1. Add all the ingredients to a blender and blend until smooth.
2. Enjoy.

PER SERVING

Calories: 656 | protein: 63g|carbs: 55g|fat: 21g

Jason'S Homemade Mass Gainer

Prep time: 5 minutes | Cook time: 5 minutes| Serves 1

- 2 scoop of chocolate whey protein powder
- 2 cups of whole milk
- ½ cup of dry rolled oats
- 1 whole banana
- 2 tbsp of organic almond butter
- 1 cup of crushed ice

1. Add all the ingredients to a blender and blend until smooth.
2. Enjoy.

PER SERVING

Calories: 970 | protein: 75g|carbs: 90g|fat: 30g

Berry Protein Shake

Prep time: 5 minutes | Cook time: 5 minutes| Serves 1

- 2 scoop of whey protein powder
- 1 cup of blueberries
- 1 cup of blackberries
- 1 cup of raspberries
- 1 cup of water
- 1 cup of ice

1. Add all the ingredients to a blender and blend until smooth.
2. Enjoy.

PER SERVING

Calories: 342 | protein: 38g|carbs: 42g|fat: 3g

Choco Coffee Energy Shake

Prep time: 5 minutes | Cook time: 5 minutes| Serves 1

- 2 scoops of chocolate protein powder
- I cup of low-fat milk
- 1 cup of water
- 1 tbsp of instant coffee

1. Add all the ingredients to a blender and blend until smooth.
2. Enjoy.

PER SERVING

Calories: 299 | protein: 42g|carbs: 14g|fat: 6g

Lean And Mean Pineapple Shake

Prep time: 5 minutes | Cook time: 5 minutes| Serves 1

- 1 cup chopped fresh pineapple
- 4 strawberries
- 1 banana
- 1 tbsp low-fat Greek yogurt
- 1 scoop of vanilla protein powder
- 1 cup of water

1. Add all the ingredients to a blender and blend until smooth.
2. Enjoy.

PER SERVING

Calories: 355 | protein: 23g|carbs: 65g|fat: 3g

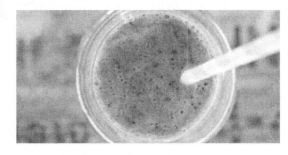

Chopped Almond Smoothie

Prep time: 5 minutes | Cook time: 5 minutes | Serves 1

- 1 1/2 cups water
- 17 chopped almonds
- 1/2 tsp coconut extract
- 1 scoop chocolate protein powder

1. Add all the ingredients to a blender and blend until smooth.
2. Enjoy.

PER SERVING

Calories: 241 | protein: 24g|carbs: 6g|fat: 13g

Breakfast Banana Shake

Prep time: 5 minutes | Cook time: 5 minutes | Serves 1

- 1 cup low-fat milk
- 1 banana
- 1 cup of rolled oats
- 2 scoops of vanilla whey protein powder

1. Add all the ingredients to a blender and blend until smooth.
2. Enjoy.

PER SERVING

Calories: 566 | protein: 59g|carbs: 69g|fat: 6g

Cinnamon And Sugar Shake

Prep time: 3 minutes | Serves 1

- 1 scoop casein protein powder, vanilla or cinnamon flavor
- 1 tablespoon milled flaxseed
- ¼ teaspoon ground cinnamon
- ¼ teaspoon vanilla extract
- 1 cup water
- 1 handful ice

1. In a blender, blend the protein powder, flaxseed, cinnamon, vanilla, water, and ice until smooth.
2. Pour into a glass and enjoy.

PER SERVING

Calories: 160 |carbs: 9g|fat: 2.2g|protein 26.5g

Vanilla Strawberry Surprise

Prep time: 5 minutes | Cook time: 5 minutes | Serves 1

- 2 scoops of vanilla protein powder
- 1 cup of ice
- 1 banana
- 4 fresh or frozen strawberries

1. Add all the ingredients to a blender and blend until smooth.
2. Enjoy.

PER SERVING

Calories: 329 | protein: 36g|carbs: 42g|fat: 2g

Banana-Nut Muffin Shake

Prep time: 3 minutes | Serves 1

- 10 raw unsalted almonds
- 1 cup unsweetened vanilla almond milk
- ½ banana
- ¼ cup whole rolled oatmeal
- 1 scoop whey isolate protein, vanilla or cinnamon flavor
- 1 handful ice

1. In a blender, blend the almonds, almond milk, banana, oatmeal, whey protein, and ice until smooth.
2. Pour into a glass and enjoy.

PER SERVING

Calories: 312|carbs: 28g|fat: 9g|protein 30g

Fresh Strawberry Shake

Prep time: 5 minutes | Cook time: 5 minutes | Serves 1

- 2 scoops of vanilla protein powder
- 1 cup of strawberries
- 2 cups of water
- 1 tbsp of flaxseed oil

1. Add all the ingredients to a blender and blend until smooth.
2. Enjoy.

PER SERVING

Calories: 303 | protein: 35g|carbs: 15g|fat: 11g

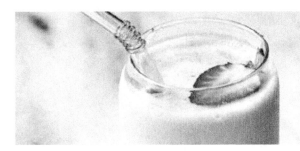
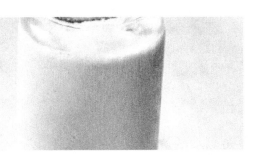

Protein Pumpkin-Spice Latte

Prep time: 3 minutes | Serves 1

- 1 cup coffee, room temperature
- 1 scoop casein, vanilla flavor
- 1 tablespoon granulated stevia
- ¼ teaspoon ground cinnamon
- ⅛ teaspoon ground nutmeg
- ¼ teaspoon pumpkin flavor extract
- 1 handful ice

1. In a blender, blend the coffee, casein, stevia, cinnamon, nutmeg, pumpkin extract, and ice until smooth.
2. Pour into a glass and enjoy.

PER SERVING

Calories: 120 |carbs: 4g|fat: 0g|protein 24g

Protein Piña Colada

Prep time: 3 minutes | Serves 1

- 1 scoop casein protein powder, vanilla flavor
- 1 cup tightly packed baby spinach
- 1 cup pineapple chunks, fresh or frozen
- 1 cup water
- ¼ cup reduced-fat unsweetened coconut milk
- 2 tablespoons granulated stevia (optional)
- 1 handful ice (if using fresh pineapple)

1. In a blender, blend the casein, spinach, pineapple, water, coconut milk, stevia, and ice (if using) until smooth.
2. Pour into a glass and enjoy.

PER SERVING

Calories:253 |carbs: 29g|fat: 10g|protein :27g

Protein Horchata

Prep time: 3 minutes | Serves 1

- 1½ cups unsweetened almond milk
- 1 scoop whey protein isolate, vanilla flavor
- 1 to 2 tablespoons granulated stevia
- ½ teaspoon ground cinnamon
- ¼ teaspoon vanilla extract

1. In a shaker cup or blender, shake or blend the almond milk, protein powder, stevia, cinnamon, and vanilla until smooth.
2. Pour into a glass and enjoy.

PER SERVING

Calories: 150 |carbs: 5g|fat: 3g|protein 25g

Chai-Banana Protein Shake

Prep time: 5 minutes, plus time to steep and chill tea | Cook time: 5 minutes| Serves 1

- 1 cup water
- 2 chai tea bags
- 1/3 cup 2% milk
- 1/3 cup 2% Greek yogurt
- 1/2 banana, preferably frozen, peeled and sliced
- 1/2 scoop vanilla protein powder
- 2 teaspoons maca powder (optional)
- 6 ice cubes
- Ground cinnamon, to taste

1. In a small pot, add water and bring to a boil over high heat. Remove from heat, add tea bags, and let tea steep for 30 minutes to fully infuse with chai flavor. Place tea in the fridge or freezer to fully chill.
2. Once tea is cool, add milk, yogurt, banana, protein powder, and (optional) maca powder into a blender. Process until smooth.
3. Pour in cold tea and blend until smooth. Add ice and continue puréeing until ice is crushed.
4. Pour shake into a glass, garnish with cinnamon, and enjoy.

PER SERVING

Calories: 243| protein: 24g| carbs: 30g|fat: 3g

Low-Carb Chocolate-Espresso Protein Shake

Prep time: 5 minutes | Cook time: 5 minutes| Serves 1

- 3/4 cup unsweetened almond milk
- 1/4 cup heavy cream
- 2 cups ice cubes
- 1 scoop chocolate protein powder
- 1 tablespoon unsweetened cocoa powder
- 1 teaspoon instant espresso powder dissolved into 2 tablespoons hot water
- 1 tablespoon granulated sugar

1. Into a blender, add almond milk, cream, ice, protein powder, cocoa powder, hot water with espresso powder, and sugar.
2. Blend ingredients until smooth. Pour smoothie into a glass to drink immediately or freeze for later enjoyment.

PER SERVING

Calories:335 | protein: 24g| carbs: 11g|fat: 23g

Wild Berry Smoothie

Prep time: 3 minutes | Serves 1

- 1 scoop whey isolate protein powder, vanilla flavor
- 1½ cups water
- ½ cup nonfat Greek yogurt
- ¼ cup blueberries, fresh or frozen
- ¼ cup raspberries, fresh or frozen
- ¼ cup strawberries, fresh or frozen
- 2 tablespoons granulated stevia
- 1 handful ice (if using fresh berries)

1. In a blender, blend the protein powder, water, yogurt, berries, stevia, and ice (if using) until smooth.
2. Pour into a glass and enjoy.

PER SERVING

Calories: 216 |carbs: 17g|fat: 1g|protein:37g

Carrot Cake Shake

Prep time 10 minutes | Cook time 5 minutes| Serves 1

- 1 cup shredded carrots
- $\frac{1}{2}$ cup unsweetened vanilla almond milk
- $\frac{1}{2}$ cup plain nonfat Greek yogurt
- 3 tbsp vanilla whey protein powder
- $\frac{1}{2}$ medium frozen banana
- $\frac{1}{8}$ tsp ground cardamom
- $\frac{1}{4}$ tsp ground ginger
- $\frac{1}{4}$ tsp ground cinnamon
- 1 tsp powdered stevia

1. Place the carrots in a microwave-safe dish, cover with a damp paper towel, and microwave on high for 1 minute. Allow to cool for 5 minutes.
2. Combine all ingredients in a blender. Blend on high for one minute. Scrape the sides of the blender with a rubber spatula, and blend on high for 1 additional minute. Transfer to a glass and serve immediately.

PER SERVING

Calories:290 |fat:1.7g|carbs: 37.2g| protein: 33.4g

Elvis Shake

Prep time 10 minutes | Cook time 5 minutes| Serves 1

- $\frac{1}{2}$ medium banana
- $\frac{1}{4}$ cup powdered peanut butter
- 1 cup unsweetened almond milk
- $\frac{1}{4}$ cup vanilla whey protein powder
- $\frac{1}{2}$ tsp vanilla extract
- $\frac{1}{2}$ tsp powdered stevia
- 1 cup crushed ice

1. Combine the banana, powdered peanut butter, almond milk, protein powder, vanilla, stevia, and ice in a blender. Blend on low for 30 seconds.
2. Scrape the sides of the blender with a rubber

spatula. Blend on high for an additional 30 seconds to 1 minute, or until the ice is crushed and the shake is smooth and creamy. Transfer to a glass and serve immediately.

PER SERVING

Calories:260 |fat:4.9g|carbs: 23g| protein: 34.1g

Orange Beet Protein Shake

Prep time: 5 minutes | Cook time: 5 minutes| Serves 2

- 2 cups water
- 2 cups beet greens
- 2 beets, peeled and diced
- 2 oranges, peeled
- 2 scoops vanilla protein powder
- Juice of 1/2 lemon

1. Into a blender, add water, greens, beets, oranges, protein powder, and lemon juice.
2. Blend the ingredients until smooth. Pour shake into 2 glasses and serve.

PER SERVING

Calories: 192| protein: 25g| carbs: 25g|fat: 0g

Key Lime Shake

Prep time 10 minutes | Cook time 5 minutes| Serves 1

- $\frac{1}{2}$ cup nonfat plain Greek yogurt
- 3 tbsp vanilla whey protein powder
- 2 tbsp lime juice
- 1 cup unsweetened vanilla coconut milk
- 2 tsp powdered stevia
- 1 cup fresh baby spinach
- $\frac{1}{2}$ cup crushed ice

1. Combine the Greek yogurt, protein powder, lime juice, coconut milk, stevia, spinach, and ice in a blender. Blend on low for 1 minute.
2. Scrape the sides of the blender with a rubber spatula. Blend on high for an additional 30 seconds to 1 minute, or until the shake is smooth and creamy. Transfer to a glass and serve immediately.

PER SERVING

Calories:222 |fat:4.6g|carbs: 14.1g| protein: 31.9g

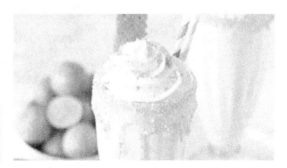

Blueberry Cheesecake Shake

Prep time 10 minutes | Cook time 5 minutes| Serves 1

- 1 cup blueberries (fresh or frozen)
- $\frac{1}{4}$ cup vanilla whey protein powder
- $\frac{1}{2}$ cup fat free plain Greek yogurt
- $\frac{1}{2}$ tsp vanilla extract
- $\frac{1}{2}$ cup unsweetened almond milk
- 1 cup crushed ice

1. Combine the blueberries, protein powder, Greek yogurt, vanilla extract, almond milk, and ice in a blender. Pulse for 15 second intervals until the ingredients are well incorporated.
2. Scrape the sides of the blender with a rubber spatula. Blend on high for 1 additional minute, or until the ice is crushed and the shake is smooth and creamy. Transfer to a glass and serve immediately.

PER SERVING

Calories:266 |fat:1.3g|carbs: 32g| protein: 32.5g

Golden Milk Shake

Prep time 10 minutes | Cook time 5 minutes| Serves 1

- 1 cup unsweetened vanilla coconut milk
- $\frac{1}{4}$ cup vanilla whey protein powder
- $\frac{1}{2}$ cup 2% low sodium cottage cheese
- $\frac{1}{2}$ tbsp coconut oil
- 1 tsp ground ginger
- $\frac{1}{2}$ tsp ground turmeric
- $\frac{1}{2}$ tsp ground cinnamon
- $\frac{1}{4}$ tsp ground black pepper
- 2 tsp powdered stevia
- $\frac{1}{2}$ cup crushed ice

1. Combine the coconut milk, protein powder, cottage cheese, coconut oil, ginger, turmeric, cinnamon, black pepper, stevia, and ice in a blender. Blend on low for 30 seconds, or until the ingredients are well incorporated.
2. Scrape the sides of the blender with a rubber spatula. Blend on high for one additional minute, or until the shake is smooth and creamy. Transfer to a glass and serve immediately.

PER SERVING

Calories:294 |fat:13.8g|carbs: 11g| protein: 34g

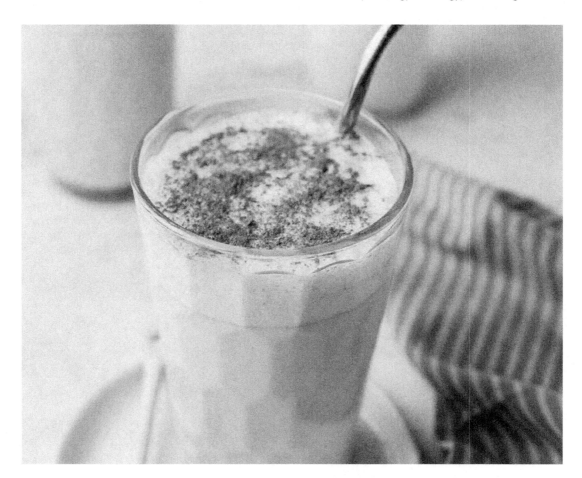

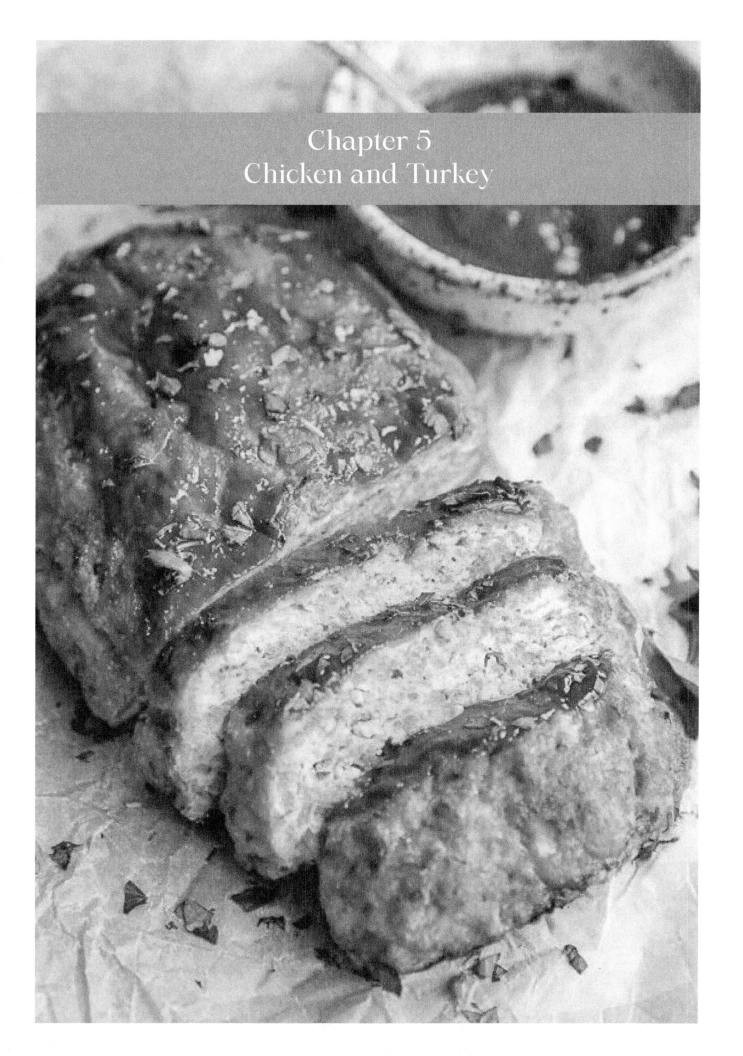

Chapter 5
Chicken and Turkey

Cashew and Spinach Basil Chicken Pasta

Prep time: 15 minutes | Cook time: 19 minutes | Serves 4

- 1½ tablespoons olive oil, divided
- 12 ounces boneless, skinless chicken breast, cut into slices
- 1 teaspoon dried basil
- 3 garlic cloves, crushed
- ½ red bell pepper, seeded and chopped
- 1 green bell pepper, seeded and chopped
- 3 tablespoons cashew pesto
- 1 cup fresh baby spinach
- 2 Roma tomatoes, chopped
- ½ cup shredded smoked low-fat cheddar cheese

1. Cook the pasta according to the package instructions. Drain and reserve ½ cup of the cooking water.
2. Heat 1 tablespoon of olive oil in large nonstick skillet over medium-high heat. Add the chicken and cook for 5 to 6 minutes. Flip over the chicken and cook until golden brown and cooked through, 4 to 6 minutes. Transfer to a plate and set aside.
3. In the same skillet, heat the remaining ½ tablespoon of oil over medium heat. Add the basil and cook, stirring, for 30 seconds. Add the garlic and cook, stirring, until lightly browned, about 30 seconds. Add the red and green bell peppers and the reserved pasta water and cook, stirring frequently, until the peppers are slightly tender, 4 to 5 minutes.
4. Add the pesto and cook, stirring, for 1 minute. Add the chicken, pasta, spinach, and tomatoes and mix well until combined. Remove the pan from the heat, sprinkle evenly with the cheese, and mix well.
5. Divide the mixture between 4 bowls and serve immediately.

PER SERVING

Calories: 481| Fat: 18 g | Protein: 34g | Sodium: 272mg | Fiber: 7 g | Carbohydrates: 49g | Sugar: 2g

Rice and Chicken and Veggie Skewers

Prep time: 10 minutes | Cook time: 30 minutes | Serves 4

- 1½ cups quick brown rice
- 2 tablespoons balsamic vinegar
- 2 tablespoons olive oil
- ⅛ teaspoon Dijon mustard
- Sea salt
- Freshly ground black pepper
- 1 pound boneless, skinless chicken breast, cut into 1-inch pieces
- 1 medium zucchini, cut into 1-inch slices
- 1 yellow bell pepper, seeded and cut into 1-inch pieces
- 1 large white onion, peeled and cut into 16 wedges

1. Cook the rice according to the package instructions.
2. Soak 12 wooden skewers in warm water for 30 minutes.
3. In a large zip-top plastic bag, mix the balsamic vinegar, olive oil, mustard, salt, and pepper. Add the chicken and seal the bag, making sure to re-

move as much air as possible. Squish the chicken around in the bag to ensure that all the pieces are evenly coated. Refrigerate for at least 30 minutes.
4. Preheat the oven to 450°F (235°C). Line 2 baking sheets with aluminum foil.
5. Place skewers on the prepared baking sheets and bake for 25 to 30 minutes, flipping the skewers after 15 minutes, or until cooked through.
6. Divide the rice between 4 plates and top with skewers of meat and vegetables.

PER SERVING

Calories: 497| Fat: 12 g | Protein: 32g | Sodium: 64mg | Fiber: 4 g | Carbohydrates: 63g | Sugar: 2g

Turkey Meatballs and Zoodles

Prep time: 10 minutes | Cook time: 25 minutes | Serves 2

- 9 ounces extra-lean ground turkey
- 1 large egg, beaten
- 1½ tablespoons bread crumbs
- ½ tablespoon dried oregano
- ½ tablespoon Italian seasoning
- 1 teaspoon garlic powder
- Sea salt
- Freshly ground black pepper
- ⅓ cup grated reduced-fat Parmesan cheese
- 3 medium zucchini, ends trimmed
- 1 tablespoon olive oil
- 1 cup low-sodium marinara sauce

1. Preheat the oven to 375°F. Line a baking sheet with parchment paper.
2. In a large bowl, mix the turkey, egg, bread crumbs, oregano, Italian seasoning, and garlic powder. Season with the salt and pepper. Using your hands, form 8 equal balls. Using your finger, create a hole in the center of each ball. Press about 1½ tablespoons of cheese into the hole and pinch the meat together to enclose the cheese completely. Place the meatballs on the prepared baking sheet and bake for 25 to 28 minutes, or until center's internal temperature is 165°F.
3. While the meatballs are baking, use a spiralizer or vegetable peeler to make noodles or ribbons from the zucchini. Pat the zucchini noodles dry to remove excess water.
4. When the meatballs are nearly cooked, heat the oil in a nonstick skillet over medium heat. Add the zucchini noodles and sauté until they are slightly soft, 3 to 4 minutes. Be careful not to overcook—they can become soggy. Transfer the noodles to a plate.
5. In the same skillet over medium heat, combine the marinara sauce and meatballs and cook until warmed through.
6. To serve, divide the noodles between 2 plates and top with the meatballs and sauce. Season with the salt and pepper, to taste.

PER SERVING

Calories: 439| Fat: 25g| Total Carbohydrates: 22g| Net Carbs: 16g| Fiber: 6g| Protein: 36g| Sodium: 451mg

Garlicky Turkey Meatballs and Zoodles

Prep time: 15 minutes | Cook time: 30 minutes | Serves 2

- 9 ounces (225g) extra-lean ground turkey
- 1 large egg, beaten
- 1½ tablespoons bread crumbs
- ½ tablespoon dried oregano
- ½ tablespoon Italian seasoning
- 1 teaspoon garlic powder
- Sea salt
- Freshly ground black pepper
- ⅓ cup grated reduced-fat Parmesan cheese
- 3 medium zucchini, ends trimmed
- 1 tablespoon olive oil
- 1 cup low-sodium marinara sauce

1. Preheat the oven to 375°F (190°C). Line a baking sheet with parchment paper.
2. In a large bowl, mix the turkey, egg, bread crumbs, oregano, Italian seasoning, and garlic powder. Season with the salt and pepper. Using your hands, form 8 equal balls. Using your finger, create a hole in the center of each ball. Press about 1½ tablespoons of cheese into the hole and pinch the meat together to enclose the cheese completely. Place the meatballs on the prepared baking sheet and bake for 25 to 28 minutes, or until center's internal temperature is 165°F (74°C).
3. While the meatballs are baking, use a spiralizer or vegetable peeler to make noodles or ribbons from the zucchini. Pat the zucchini noodles dry to remove excess water.
4. When the meatballs are nearly cooked, heat the oil in a nonstick skillet over medium heat. Add the zucchini noodles and sauté until they are slightly soft, 3 to 4 minutes. Be careful not to overcook—they can become soggy. Transfer the noodles to a plate.
5. In the same skillet over medium heat, combine the marinara sauce and meatballs and cook until warmed through.
6. To serve, divide the noodles between 2 plates and top with the meatballs and sauce. Season with the salt and pepper, to taste.

PER SERVING

Calories: 439| Fat: 25 g | Protein: 36g | Sodium: 451mg | Fiber: 6 g | Carbohydrates: 36g | Sugar: 3g

Spinach and Garlic Chicken Burger

Prep time: 15 minutes | Cook time: 15 minutes | Serves 2

- 1 pound (454g) extra-lean ground chicken
- 1 large egg
- ¼ small white onion, diced
- 1 garlic clove, minced
- 1 tablespoon chopped fresh cilantro
- 1 tablespoon Worcestershire sauce
- 1 tablespoon olive oil
- ½ cup shredded reduced-fat cheddar cheese
- 4 whole-grain buns
- 4 tomatoes, thickly sliced
- 1 cup fresh baby spinach

1. In a large bowl, mix the chicken, egg, onion, garlic, cilantro, and Worcestershire sauce. Form the mixture into 4 equal patties and place on a plate.
2. Heat the olive oil in a nonstick skillet over medium-high heat. Cook the patties in the skillet for 5 to 6 minutes. Flip the patties over and cook for 4 minutes. Sprinkle them with the cheese, cover, and cook until the patties are cooked through, 1 to 2 more minutes. Transfer the burgers to a plate and set aside.
3. Add the buns, cut-side down, to the skillet and cook until lightly browned, 3 minutes.
4. To serve, place a burger on each bun and top with the slices of tomatoes and the spinach.

PER SERVING

Calories 378| Fat 18g| Protein 30g| Sodium 460mg| | Fiber 3g| Carbohydrates 26g| Sugar 6g|

Pulled-Chicken BBQ Sandwiches

Prep time: 5 minutes | Cook time: 10 minutes| Serves 1

- 4 ounces shredded slow-cooked chicken
- 2 tablespoons barbecue sauce (or any other sauce of your choice)
- 1 whole-wheat hamburger bun

1. In a medium bowl, mix chicken and sauce until chicken is coated completely. (It's best if chicken is heated.)
2. Place chicken on sandwich bun and serve.

PER SERVING

Calories: 316 | Fat: 3g | Protein: 29g | Sodium: 1,003mg | Fiber: 4g | Carbohydrates: 43g | Sugar: 14g

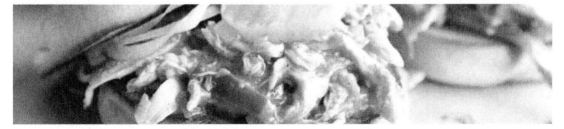

Balsamic Chicken and Veggie Skewers

Prep time: 10 minutes, plus 30 minutes marinating | Cook time: 50 minutes | Serves 4

- 1½ cups quick brown rice
- 2 tablespoons balsamic vinegar
- 2 tablespoons olive oil
- ⅛ teaspoon Dijon mustard
- Sea salt
- Freshly ground black pepper
- 1 pound boneless, skinless chicken breast, cut into 1-inch pieces
- 1 medium zucchini, cut into 1-inch slices
- 1 yellow bell pepper, seeded and cut into 1-inch pieces
- 1 large white onion, peeled and cut into 16 wedges

1. Cook the rice according to the package instructions.
2. Soak 12 wooden skewers in warm water for 30 minutes.
3. In a large zip-top plastic bag, mix the balsamic vinegar, olive oil, mustard, salt, and pepper. Add the chicken and seal the bag, making sure to remove as much air as possible. Squish the chicken around in the bag to ensure that all the pieces are evenly coated. Refrigerate for at least 30 minutes.
4. Preheat the oven to 450°F. Line 2 baking sheets with aluminum foil.
5. Remove the chicken from the marinade and discard the marinade. Thread the chicken, zucchini, bell pepper, and onion on the skewers.
6. Place skewers on the prepared baking sheets and bake for 25 to 30 minutes, flipping the skewers after 15 minutes, or until cooked through.
7. Divide the rice between 4 plates and top with skewers of meat and vegetables.

PER SERVING

Calories: 497 | Fat: 12g | Total Carbohydrates: 63g | Net Carbs: 59g | Fiber: 4g | Protein: 32g | Sodium: 64mg

Oregano and Cucumber-Chicken Wraps

Prep time: 15 minutes | Cook time: 13 minutes | Serves 2

- ⅔ cups plain nonfat Greek yogurt
- ¼ cup shredded cucumber
- 2 garlic cloves, finely minced, divided
- 1 tablespoon hemp hearts
- ½ tablespoon freshly squeezed lemon juice
- Sea salt
- Freshly ground black pepper
- ½ tablespoon olive oil
- 6 ounces boneless, skinless chicken breast, cut into thin slices
- 1½ teaspoons dried oregano
- 2 (10-inch) 100% whole wheat wraps
- 2 cups mixed greens
- 2 tablespoons crumbled reduced-fat feta cheese

1. In a medium bowl, mix the Greek yogurt, cucumber, half the garlic, the hemp hearts, and the lemon juice. Season with salt and pepper to taste. Set aside.
2. Heat the olive oil in a large nonstick skillet over medium-high heat. Add the remaining half of the garlic and sauté for 1 minute. Add the chicken and cook, stirring frequently, until golden brown and cooked through, 8 to 12 minutes. Add the oregano and season with salt and pepper to taste.
3. To assemble the wraps: Spread each wrap with the cucumber yogurt and top with the mixed greens, chicken, and feta. Wrap up and enjoy.

PER SERVING

Calories: 434 | Fat: 12 g | Protein: 36g | Sodium: 669mg | Fiber: 3 g | Carbohydrates: 44g | Sugar: 2g

Feta Turkey Burgers

Prep time: 5 minutes | Cook time: 15 minutes | Serves 4

- 1 tablespoon (15ml) extra-virgin olive oil or avocado oil
- ½ medium onion (47g), chopped
- 1 cup (30g) chopped baby spinach
- 2 garlic cloves (10g), minced
- 1 pound (453g) lean ground turkey
- ½ cup (75g) crumbled feta cheese
- 2 tablespoons (11g) chopped fresh basil
- 1 teaspoon (1.5g) dried oregano
- ½ teaspoon (3g) sea salt
- ¼ teaspoon (0.5g) freshly ground black pepper
- Nonstick cooking spray

1. In a medium nonstick skillet over medium-high heat, heat the olive oil. Add the onion and sauté for about 5 minutes, or until translucent. Add the spinach and garlic and sauté until the spinach is wilted, about 3 more minutes.
2. Transfer to a large bowl and add the turkey, feta, basil, oregano, salt, and pepper.
3. Lightly spray the palms of your hands with non-stick spray, and use your hands to mix everything together until well combined. Form into 4 equal-size patties.
4. Heat a large nonstick skillet over medium-high heat. Spray both sides of each patty lightly with the cooking spray, then place in the pan. Cook for about 4 minutes on each side, until cooked through and the internal temperature reads 165°F.
5. Into each of 4 airtight storage containers, place 1 burger and seal.

PER SERVING

Calories: 239 | Fat: 14g | Protein: 27g | Total Carbs: 3g | Net Carbs: 2g | Fiber: 1g | Sugar: 1g | Sodium: 593mg

Garlic-Chicken Burger

Prep time: 10 minutes | Cook time: 15 minutes| Serves 4

- 1 pound extra-lean ground chicken
- 1 large egg
- ¼ small white onion, diced
- 1 garlic clove, minced
- 1 tablespoon chopped fresh cilantro
- 1 tablespoon Worcestershire sauce
- 1 tablespoon olive oil
- ½ cup shredded reduced-fat cheddar cheese
- 4 whole-grain buns
- 4 tomatoes, thickly sliced
- 1 cup fresh baby spinach

1. In a large bowl, mix the chicken, egg, onion, garlic, cilantro, and Worcestershire sauce. Form the mixture into 4 equal patties and place on a plate.
2. Heat the olive oil in a nonstick skillet over medium-high heat. Cook the patties in the skillet for 5 to 6 minutes. Flip the patties over and cook for 4 minutes. Sprinkle them with the cheese, cover, and cook until the patties are cooked through, 1 to 2 more minutes. Transfer the burgers to a plate and set aside.
3. Add the buns, cut-side down, to the skillet and cook until lightly browned, 3 minutes.
4. To serve, place a burger on each bun and top with the slices of tomatoes and the spinach.

PER SERVING

Calories: 378| Fat: 18g| Total Carbohydrates: 26g| Net Carbs: 23g| Fiber: 3g| Protein: 30g| Sodium: 460mg

Beer Can Chicken

Prep time: 5 minutes | Cook time: 1 hour 20 minutes|Serves 4

- 1 (3–5-pound) whole medium chicken
- 2 tablespoons olive oil or other vegetable oil
- 1 tablespoon salt
- 1 tablespoon freshly ground black pepper
- 2 tablespoons chopped fresh thyme leaves or 1 tablespoon dried thyme
- 1 (12-ounce) can beer, room temperature

1. Prepare grill for indirect heat cooking by turning on only one side of burners to medium-high and allowing entire grill to heat to 350°F.
2. Remove innards from chicken and discard. Brush chicken lightly with oil.
3. In a small bowl, combine salt, pepper, and thyme and cover chicken with rub mixture.
4. Open beer, pour out half, and use a knife to carefully cut openings into the top half of the open can. Carefully stand the chicken upright, so that the can is inside its cavity, and place the entire chicken on the cool side of the grill, making sure it stands up on its own. Cover grill.
5. Do not open the grill for at least 1 hour, then check every 15 minutes until fully cooked. A thermometer inserted should read 160–165°F when fully cooked.
6. Remove, allow to rest at least 10 minutes, then cut and serve.

PER SERVING

Calories: 368 | Fat: 14g | Protein: 49g | Sodium: 144mg | Fiber: 1g | Carbohydrates: 4g | Sugar: 0g

Scallions and Feta Stuffed Chicken

Prep time: 15 minutes | Cook time: 33 minutes | Serves 4

- 3 teaspoons olive oil, divided
- ⅓ cup finely chopped scallions
- 2 garlic cloves, minced
- 3 cups finely chopped spinach
- ¾ cup crumbled reduced-fat feta cheese
- 2 tablespoons crushed cashews
- 2 tablespoons minced fresh parsley
- ¼ teaspoon chili powder
- ½ teaspoon sea salt, divided
- 4 (4-ounce (113g)) boneless, skinless chicken breasts

1. Preheat the oven to 350°F (180°C). Line a baking sheet with aluminum foil.
2. Heat 1 teaspoon of olive oil in a large nonstick skillet over medium heat. Add the scallions and garlic and sauté for 1 minute. Add the spinach and cook, stirring, until it starts to wilt, 1 to 2 minutes. Remove from the heat. Add the feta, cashews, parsley, chili powder, and ¼ teaspoon of salt. Set aside.
3. Cut a 2-inch pocket in the center of each chicken breast and divide the spinach mixture between the 4 chicken breasts.
4. Using a basting brush, spread the remaining 2 teaspoons of olive oil over the chicken. Season with the remaining ¼ teaspoon of salt and pepper. Bake stuffed breasts on the prepared baking sheet for 25 to 30 minutes, or until the chicken is no longer pink and the juices run clear. Serve immediately.

PER SERVING

Calories 275| Fat 14g| Protein 31g| Sodium 567mg| | Fiber 1g| Carbohydrates 4g| Sugar 1g|

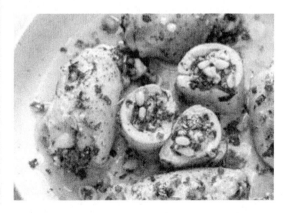

Turkey and Spinach Focaccia Sandwich

Prep time: 5 minutes | Cook time: 10 minutes| Serves 2

- 2 tablespoons low-fat mayonnaise
- 2 tablespoons chopped fresh basil
- 2 tablespoons sun-dried tomatoes
- ¼ teaspoon crushed red pepper
- 8 ounces sliced turkey
- 1 cup spinach leaves
- 4 slices focaccia bread

1. In a small bowl, mix mayonnaise, basil, tomatoes, and crushed red pepper. Divide the mixture in half.
2. Build sandwiches by layering the spread, turkey, and spinach leaves on two slices focaccia, and then topping with two slices.

PER SERVING

Calories: 421 | Fat: 13g | Protein: 25g | Sodium: 1,679mg | Fiber: 1g | Carbohydrates: 52g | Sugar: 3g

Maple-Ginger Chicken Stir-Fry

Prep time: 10 minutes | Cook time: 40 minutes| Serves 2

- ¾ cup quick brown rice
- 3 tablespoons low-sodium soy sauce
- 2 tablespoons maple syrup
- 3 tablespoons water
- 1 tablespoon olive oil, divided
- 2 large carrots, peeled and diced
- 1 green bell pepper, seeded and diced
- 1½ teaspoons minced garlic
- 1 teaspoon minced ginger
- 10 ounces boneless, skinless chicken breast, cut into 1-inch pieces
- Sea salt
- Freshly ground black pepper

1. Cook the rice according to the package instructions.
2. In a small bowl, mix soy sauce, maple syrup, and water. Set aside.
3. Heat ½ tablespoon of olive oil in a large nonstick skillet over medium heat. Add the carrots and cook, stirring, for 4 to 5 minutes. Add the bell pepper to cook until the carrots are tender and slightly soft, 3 to 5 minutes. Transfer the mixture to a bowl.
4. In the same skillet, heat the remaining ½ tablespoon of oil over medium-high heat. Add the garlic and ginger and sauté for 1 minute. Add the chicken and cook, stirring frequently, until golden brown and cooked through, 8 to 12 minutes. Reduce the heat, add the vegetable mixture and the sauce, and mix well. Season with salt and pepper to taste.
5. Divide the recipe between 2 bowls and top with the chicken and vegetable mixture. Serve immediately.

PER SERVING

Calories: 597| Fat: 13g| Total Carbohydrates: 79g| Net Carbs: 73g| Fiber: 6g| Protein: 41g| Sodium: 887mg

Basil-Chicken Pasta

Prep time: 15 minutes | Cook time: 25 minutes| Serves 4

- 8 ounces whole wheat penne
- 1½ tablespoons olive oil, divided
- 12 ounces boneless, skinless chicken breast, cut into slices
- 1 teaspoon dried basil
- 3 garlic cloves, crushed
- ½ red bell pepper, seeded and chopped
- 1 green bell pepper, seeded and chopped
- 3 tablespoons cashew pesto
- 1 cup fresh baby spinach
- 2 Roma tomatoes, chopped
- ½ cup shredded smoked low-fat cheddar cheese

1. Cook the pasta according to the package instructions. Drain and reserve ½ cup of the cooking water.
2. Heat 1 tablespoon of olive oil in large nonstick skillet over medium-high heat. Add the chicken and cook for 5 to 6 minutes. Flip over the chicken and cook until golden brown and cooked through, 4 to 6 minutes. Transfer to a plate and set aside.
3. In the same skillet, heat the remaining ½ tablespoon of oil over medium heat. Add the basil and cook, stirring, for 30 seconds. Add the garlic and cook, stirring, until lightly browned, about 30 seconds. Add the red and green bell peppers and the reserved pasta water and cook, stirring frequently, until the peppers are slightly tender, 4 to 5 minutes.
4. Add the pesto and cook, stirring, for 1 minute. Add the chicken, pasta, spinach, and tomatoes and mix well until combined. Remove the pan from the heat, sprinkle evenly with the cheese, and mix well.
5. Divide the mixture between 4 bowls and serve immediately.

PER SERVING

Calories: 481| Fat: 18g| Total Carbohydrates: 49g| Net Carbs: 42g| Fiber: 7g| Protein: 34g| Sodium: 272mg

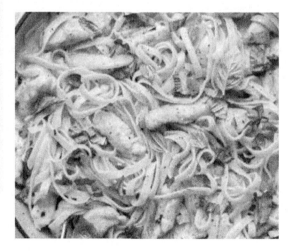

Chicken with Mango Salsa

Prep time: 10 minutes | Cook time: 25 minutes| Serves 4

- 1 tablespoon olive oil
- 4 (4-ounce) boneless, skinless chicken breasts
- ½ teaspoon sea salt
- ¼ teaspoon freshly ground black pepper
- 1 avocado, pitted, peeled, and diced
- 1 cup diced fresh or frozen mango
- 1 garlic clove, minced
- ¼ cup minced red onion
- ¼ cup chopped fresh cilantro
- 2 tablespoons lime juice
- 1 teaspoon olive oil
- 8 cups mixed greens

1. Preheat the oven to 400°F. Line a baking sheet with aluminum foil.
2. Using a basting brush, spread the olive oil over the chicken and season with the salt and pepper. Arrange the chicken on the prepared baking sheet and bake for 20 to 25 minutes, or until cooked through.
3. While the chicken bakes, in a large bowl, mix the avocado, mango, garlic, red onion, and cilantro. Add the lime juice and oil and stir until combined. Cover with plastic wrap and refrigerate until ready to serve.
4. Place a chicken breast on each of 4 plates. Divide the mixed greens between the plates and top with mango salsa.

PER SERVING

Calories: 313| Fat: 16g| Total Carbohydrates: 16g| Net Carbs: 10g| Fiber: 6g| Protein: 29g| Sodium: 292mg

Southwestern Chicken Wraps

Prep time: 15 minutes | Cook time: 30 minutes| Serves 4

- 1½ cups (210g) chopped boneless, skinless chicken
- 1 teaspoon (2.4g) onion powder
- 1 teaspoon (2.4g) garlic powder
- 1 teaspoon (2.4g) ground cumin
- 1 teaspoon (2.4g) chili powder
- Sea salt
- Freshly ground black pepper
- 1 tablespoon (15ml) extra-virgin olive oil
- 1 red bell pepper (150g), cut into strips
- ½ red onion (75g), diced
- 1 tomato (100g), diced
- ½ cup (40g) cooked black beans
- 6 tablespoons (85g) sliced black olives
- 1 jalapeño (15g), seeded and minced
- ½ bunch cilantro (27g), chopped
- 4 (10-inch) tortillas (220g)
- ¼ cup (120g) reduced-fat sour cream (5%), divided
- ¼ cup (30g) shredded Monterey Jack cheese, divided
- ¼ cup (30g) crumbled feta, divided

1. Heat a grill to medium-high or preheat the broiler

to high.
2. In a medium bowl, combine the chicken with the onion powder, garlic powder, cumin, and chili powder. Season with salt and pepper. Grill for 7 to 10 minutes on each side, or broil on a broiler pan 6 inches from the heat for 10 minutes on each side, until the juices run clear. Let cool completely, and cut into strips.
3. In a medium skillet over medium heat, heat the olive oil. Add the red bell pepper, onion, and tomato and cook for 3 to 4 minutes, or until tender.
4. Add the chicken, beans, olives, jalapeño, and cilantro and cook until warmed through and well combined, a few minutes more.
5. To make each wrap, place each tortilla on a cutting board and sprinkle with one-quarter of the filling.
6. Roll the tortilla around the ingredients tightly enough so the wrap will hold its shape. Repeat with the remaining tortillas.
7. Into each of 4 airtight storage containers, place 1 tortilla and top with 1 tablespoon of sour cream, 1 tablespoon of Monterey Jack cheese, and 1 tablespoon of feta and seal.

PER SERVING

Calories: 442| Fat: 15g| Protein: 28g| Total Carbs: 50g| Net Carbs: 41g| Fiber: 9g| Sugar: 5g| Sodium: 898mg

Apple-Roasted Whole Chicken

Prep time 10 minutes | Cook time 65 minutes| Serves 8

- 1 tsp salt
- 1 tsp garlic powder
- 1 tsp ground black pepper
- 1 small chicken, approximately 2½ to 3lbs (1.2 to 1.4kg), giblets removed
- 1 medium Granny Smith apple
- Coconut oil cooking spray

1. Preheat the oven to 350°F (177°C). Make the rub by combining the salt, garlic powder, and black pepper in a small bowl.
2. Place the chicken in a large roasting pan. Insert the apple into the cavity, and season the outside of the chicken with half of the rub. Place the chicken in the oven and roast for 45 minutes.
3. After 45 minutes, increase the oven temperature to 400°F (204°C). Remove the chicken from the oven, lightly spray with coconut oil spray, and season with the remaining rub.
4. Bake for an additional 15 minutes, or until the internal temperature reaches 165°F (74°C) and the juices run clear when the chicken is pierced with a sharp knife. Slice and serve hot.

PER SERVING

Calories:151 |fat:4.2g|carbs: 0g| protein: 26.4g

Cucumber-Chicken Wraps

Prep time: 10 minutes | Cook time: 15 minutes| Serves 2

- ⅔ cups plain nonfat Greek yogurt
- ¼ cup shredded cucumber
- 2 garlic cloves, finely minced, divided
- 1 tablespoon hemp hearts
- ½ tablespoon freshly squeezed lemon juice
- Sea salt
- Freshly ground black pepper
- ½ tablespoon olive oil
- 6 ounces boneless, skinless chicken breast, cut into thin slices
- 1½ teaspoons dried oregano
- 2 (10-inch) 100% whole wheat wraps
- 2 cups mixed greens
- 2 tablespoons crumbled reduced-fat feta cheese

1. In a medium bowl, mix the Greek yogurt, cucumber, half the garlic, the hemp hearts, and the lemon juice. Season with salt and pepper to taste. Set aside.
2. Heat the olive oil in a large nonstick skillet over medium-high heat. Add the remaining half of the garlic and sauté for 1 minute. Add the chicken and cook, stirring frequently, until golden brown and cooked through, 8 to 12 minutes. Add the oregano and season with salt and pepper to taste.
3. To assemble the wraps: Spread each wrap with the cucumber yogurt and top with the mixed greens, chicken, and feta. Wrap up and enjoy.

PER SERVING

Calories: 434| Fat: 12g| Total Carbohydrates: 44g| Net Carbs: 41g| Fiber: 3g| Protein: 36g| Sodium: 669mg

Chicken Parmesan

Prep time: 10 minutes | Cook time: 45 minutes| Serves 4

- 1½ cups quinoa
- Nonstick cooking spray
- 1 cup bread crumbs
- 1 tablespoon dried oregano
- 1 teaspoon smoked paprika
- ¼ cup grated reduced-fat Parmesan cheese
- 1 large egg
- 2 large egg whites
- 2 tablespoons all-purpose flour
- 4 (4½-ounce) boneless, skinless chicken breasts, each halved lengthwise
- 1 cup low-sodium marinara sauce
- ¼ cup shredded reduced-fat mozzarella cheese
- 8 cups mixed greens

1. Make the quinoa according to the package instructions.
2. Preheat the oven to 450°F. Lightly spray a baking sheet with nonstick cooking spray.
3. In a shallow dish, combine the bread crumbs, oregano, paprika, and Parmesan cheese. Set aside. In another shallow dish, beat together the egg and egg whites. Set aside.
4. Sprinkle the flour over the chicken breasts, making sure both sides are lightly coated.
5. Using one hand, dip a chicken breast in the egg mixture| using the other hand, press the egg-coated chicken breast into the bread crumb mixture. Place the chicken on the baking sheet. Repeat with the remaining chicken. Sprinkle any remaining bread crumb mixture over the chicken breasts.
6. Bake for 25 minutes. Pour ¼ cup of marinara sauce over each chicken breast and top each with 1 tablespoon of mozzarella cheese. Bake for 3 to 5 minutes more, or until the cheese is melted.
7. Divide the quinoa among 4 bowls. Top with the greens and the chicken. Serve hot.

PER SERVING

Calories: 568| Fat: 12g| Total Carbohydrates: 65g| Net Carbs: 57g| Fiber: 8g| Protein: 49g| Sodium: 394mg

Cashew And Feta Stuffed Chicken

Prep time: 15 minutes | Cook time: 30 minutes| Serves 4

- 3 teaspoons olive oil, divided
- ⅓ cup finely chopped scallions
- 2 garlic cloves, minced
- 3 cups finely chopped spinach
- ¾ cup crumbled reduced-fat feta cheese
- 2 tablespoons crushed cashews
- 2 tablespoons minced fresh parsley
- ¼ teaspoon chili powder
- ½ teaspoon sea salt, divided
- 4 (4-ounce) boneless, skinless chicken breasts

1. Preheat the oven to 350°F. Line a baking sheet with aluminum foil.
2. Heat 1 teaspoon of olive oil in a large nonstick skillet over medium heat. Add the scallions and garlic and sauté for 1 minute. Add the spinach and cook, stirring, until it starts to wilt, 1 to 2 minutes. Remove from the heat. Add the feta, cashews, parsley, chili powder, and ¼ teaspoon of salt. Set aside.
3. Cut a 2-inch pocket in the center of each chicken breast and divide the spinach mixture between the 4 chicken breasts.
4. Using a basting brush, spread the remaining 2 teaspoons of olive oil over the chicken. Season with the remaining ¼ teaspoon of salt and pepper. Bake stuffed breasts on the prepared baking sheet for 25 to 30 minutes, or until the chicken is no longer pink and the juices run clear. Serve immediately.

PER SERVING

Calories: 275| Fat: 14g| Total Carbohydrates: 4g| Net Carbs: 3g| Fiber: 1g| Protein: 31g| Sodium: 567mg

Pesto Chicken

Prep time: 5 minutes | Cook time: 25 minutes| Serves 4

- 1 pound boneless, skinless chicken breasts
- ½ teaspoon sea salt
- ¼ teaspoon freshly ground black pepper
- ¼ cup reduced-fat French onion dip
- ¾ cup nonfat plain Greek yogurt
- 2 tablespoons olive oil
- 2 garlic cloves, minced
- 2 tablespoons cashew pesto
- 1 cup halved cherry tomatoes
- ½ cup grated reduced-fat Parmesan cheese
- ⅛ cup thinly sliced fresh basil

1. Season the chicken with salt and pepper and set it aside on a plate.
2. In a small bowl, mix the French onion dip and Greek yogurt. Set aside.
3. Heat the olive oil in a nonstick skillet over medium-high heat. Add the garlic and cook for 1 minute. Add the chicken and cook for 5 to 6 minutes. Flip over the chicken and cook for 4 to 6 minutes. Add the pesto and continue to cook until browned and cooked through, another 1 to 2 minutes. Add the yogurt mixture and mix well. Increase the heat to high and bring to a boil.
4. Reduce the heat to medium, add the tomatoes, and cook until they soften, about 2 to 3 minutes. Reduce the heat to medium-low and simmer for 4 to 5 minutes. Top with the Parmesan cheese.
5. Place the chicken on a serving plate and garnish with the basil.

PER SERVING

Calories: 361| Fat: 20g| Total Carbohydrates: 11g| Net Carbs: 10g| Fiber: 1g| Protein: 34g| Sodium: 834mg

Pan-Seared Chicken Breasts

Prep time 10 minutes, plus 4 hours | Cook time 25 minutes| Serves 8

- 2 cups water
- 1 tbsp apple cider vinegar
- 2 tbsp sriracha hot chili sauce
- 1 tbsp course ground mustard
- ½ tsp ground black pepper
- 2 tbsp salt
- 1 tsp garlic powder
- 2lbs (900g) boneless, skinless chicken breasts

1. Preheat the oven to 400°F (204°C). Make the brine by combining the water, vinegar, sriracha sauce, mustard, black pepper, salt, and garlic powder in a large glass bowl. Mix well to combine.
2. Add the chicken breasts to the bowl, ensuring the brine covers the chicken completely. (Add more water to cover the chicken, if needed.) Tightly cover the bowl with plastic wrap and place in the refrigerator to brine for a minimum of 4 hours (or up to 12 hours).
3. Spray a large cast iron grill pan with coconut oil cooking spray and preheat over medium-high heat. Remove the chicken from the brine and rinse under cool water to remove any excess salt.
4. Place the chicken on the pre-heated grill pan. Sear for 3 to 4 minutes per side, then place in the oven to bake for an additional 8 to 10 minutes. The chicken is done when the juices run clear and the internal temperature reaches 165°F (74°C).

PER SERVING

Calories:140 |fat:3g|carbs: 0g| protein: 27g

Stuffed Florentine Chicken Breasts

Prep time 10 minutes | Cook time 25 minutes| Serves 4

- 3 boneless, skinless chicken breasts, or approximately 1lb (450g)
- ½ tsp salt
- ½ tsp ground black pepper
- ½ tsp garlic powder
- ½ cup chopped sun-dried tomatoes
- ½ cup chopped fresh baby spinach
- ½ cup light shredded mozzarella cheese

1. Preheat oven to 350°F (177°C). Lightly spray a medium cast iron skillet with non-stick cooking spray and place over medium-high heat.
2. Add the chicken breasts to the skillet and season with the salt, pepper, and garlic powder. Cook for 1 to 2 minutes per side, or until lightly browned.
3. Remove the skillet from the heat and allow the breasts to rest in the skillet for 5 minutes. Once the breasts are cool enough to handle, transfer to a cutting board and create pockets for the fillings by slicing halfway through each breast lengthwise, being careful not to slice completely through the breasts.
4. Stuff each breast with equal amounts of the spinach, tomatoes, and cheese, and secure by inserting a toothpick through each breast. Transfer the breasts back to the skillet and bake for 20 minutes. The chicken is done when the juices run clear and the internal temperature reaches 165°F (74°C). Serve hot.

PER SERVING

Calories:193 |fat:5g|carbs: 7g| protein: 30g

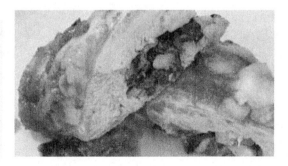

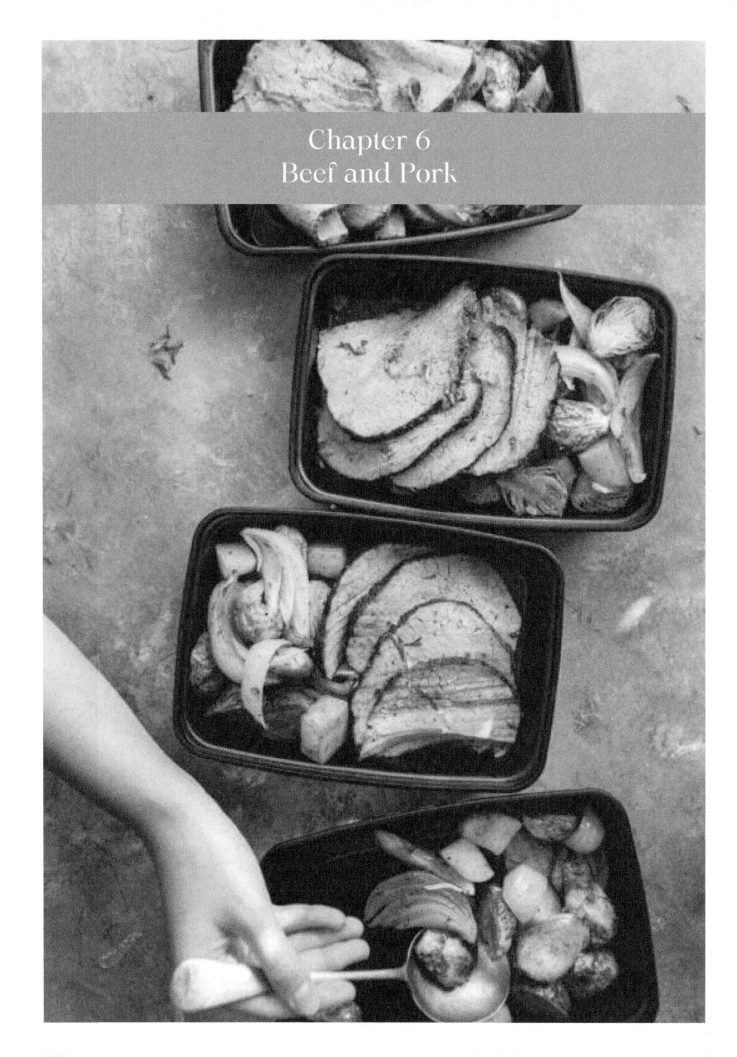

Chapter 6
Beef and Pork

Garlicky Steak and Bell Pepper Fajitas

Prep time: 15 minutes | Cook time: 20 minutes | Serves 4

- 12 ounces (340g) top sirloin steak, cut into thin slices
- 2 teaspoons paprika
- 1 teaspoon ground cumin
- ½ teaspoon garlic powder
- ½ teaspoon freshly ground black pepper
- ½ teaspoon sea salt
- 1½ tablespoons olive oil, divided
- 1 red bell pepper, seeded and thinly sliced
- 1 green bell pepper, seeded and thinly sliced
- 1 medium white onion, thinly sliced
- 4 (8-inch) whole wheat tortillas
- ½ cup fresh salsa

1. In a large bowl, toss the steak with the paprika, cumin, garlic powder, pepper, and salt until evenly coated.
2. Heat 1 tablespoon of olive oil in a large nonstick skillet over medium-high heat. Add the steak and cook, stirring frequently, until browned, 8 to 10 minutes. Transfer to a plate and set aside.
3. In the same skillet, heat the remaining ½ table-spoon of oil over medium heat. Add the red and green bell peppers and cook, stirring frequently, until tender, 4 to 5 minutes. Add the onion and continue to cook until the onion is soft, 3 to 5 minutes. Add the steak to the skillet and stir until combined. Transfer the mixture to the plate and set aside.
4. Wipe out the skillet with paper towels. Warm up the tortillas in a skillet over medium-high heat.
5. Divide the fajita filling equally between the tortillas. Top with the salsa and serve.

PER SERVING

Calories: 375 | Fat: 19 g | Protein: 23 g | Sodium: 722 mg | Fiber: 7 g | Carbohydrates: 28 g | Sugar: 1 g

Limey Beef Tacos on A Stick

Prep time: 15 minutes | Cook time: 10 minutes | Serves 4

- 1 small white onion, chopped
- Juice of 1 lime
- 1 teaspoon ground cumin
- 1 teaspoon chili powder
- ½ teaspoon garlic powder
- ¼ teaspoon sea salt
- ¼ teaspoon freshly ground black pepper
- 12 ounces beef sirloin tips, cut into 1-inch cubes
- Nonstick cooking spray
- 1 red bell pepper, seeded and cut into 1-inch pieces
- 1 large white onion, peeled and cut into 8 wedges

1. In a food processor, combine the onion, lime juice, cumin, chili powder, garlic powder, salt, and pepper and puree until smooth.
2. Transfer the mixture to a large zip-top plastic bag. Add the sirloin tips, seal, and use your hands

to squish around the beef so it's evenly coated in the marinade. Refrigerate for at least 1 hour.
3. Preheat the broiler. Spray the broiler rack with nonstick cooking spray. Remove the beef from the plastic bag and discard the marinade. Thread the beef, pepper, and onion alternately onto 8 to 12 metal skewers.
4. Place the skewers on the broiler rack and broil for 5 minutes. Turn over the skewers and broil for another 4 to 5 minutes, or until the beef is cooked through.

PER SERVING

Calories: 149 | Fat: 4 g | Protein: 19 g | Sodium: 186 mg | Fiber: 2 g | Carbohydrates: 9 g | Sugar: 3 g

Rice with Orange-Ginger Beef

Prep time: 15 minutes | Cook time: 28 minutes | Serves 4

- 1½ cups quick brown rice
- ⅓ cup freshly squeezed orange juice, no pulp
- 4 garlic cloves, minced, divided
- 1 teaspoon minced ginger
- 2 tablespoons low-sodium soy sauce
- 1 teaspoon corn starch
- 2 teaspoons water
- 2 tablespoons olive oil, divided
- 12 ounces top sirloin steak, thinly sliced
- 1 cup sliced carrots cut into ¼-inch pieces
- 1 red bell pepper, seeded and thinly sliced
- 1 green bell pepper, seeded and thinly sliced
- Sea salt
- Freshly ground black pepper

1. Cook the rice according to the package instructions. Set aside.
2. To make the marinade, in a small saucepan, combine the orange juice, half the garlic, the ginger, and the soy sauce, and bring it to a boil over medium-high heat.
3. In a small bowl, mix the cornstarch and water. Add the mixture to the saucepan, lower the heat to low, and stir until combined. Cook, stirring occasionally, until the marinade thickens, 6 to 8 minutes. Set aside.
4. Heat 1 tablespoon of the oil in a large nonstick skillet over medium-high heat. Add the steak and cook, stirring frequently, until browned, 5 to 8 minutes. Transfer to a plate.
5. In the same skillet, heat the remaining 1 table-spoon of oil. Add the remaining garlic and sauté for 1 minute. Add the carrots and cook for 4 to 5 minutes. Add the red and green bell peppers and cook until tender, 4 to 6 minutes.
6. Add the steak and the sauce and mix well.
7. Divide the rice between 4 plates. Top with the steak, including the sauce. Add salt and pepper to taste and serve.

PER SERVING

Calories: 528 | Fat: 18 g | Protein: 25 g | Sodium: 329 mg | Fiber: 5 g | Carbohydrates: 25 g | Sugar: 3 g

Brawny Beef Sandwiches

Prep time: 5 minutes | Cook time: 5 minutes| Serves 1

- 4 slices of deli beef
- 4 slices of whole-wheat bread
- 2 tsp of mustard
- Handful of baby spinach leaves
- 1/2 a sliced cucumber
- A pinch of black pepper

1. Get 2 slices of bread.
2. Add 2 slices of deli beef, 1 tsp of mustard, ½ a sliced cucumber, spinach and a pinch of black pepper to the slice and make a sandwich.
3. Repeat the process with the rest of the ingredients.

PER SERVING

Calories: 545 | protein: 43g|carbs: 64g|fat: 10g

Power Pork Fruit Tray

Prep time: 5 minutes | Cook time: 25 minutes| Serves 4

- 4 pork steaks
- 1 tbsp olive oil
- 2 diced red onions
- 2 chopped large pears
- 3 sprigs of rosemary
- 2oz diced blue cheese
- 1 diced courgette
- A pinch of salt and pepper
- Handful of pine nuts

1. Get a large pan and heat the olive oil on a medium heat.
2. Add the courgette, red onions, chopped pears, salt and pepper.
3. Fry for around 6 minutes until the veg starts to caramelise.
4. Pre-heat the Grill.
5. Get a cooking tray and transfer the ingredients along with the rosemary sprigs to the tray. Sprinkle some salt and pepper over the pork steaks and place them in the tray.
6. Place the tray in the oven and grill for around 10-15 minutes or until cooked right through, turning the pork steaks half way through. Add the cheese and pine nuts and let the cheese melt for a further 4-5 minutes.
7. Plate up and serve.

PER SERVING

Calories: 335 | protein: 42g|carbs: 12g|fat: 14g

Butter and Thyme Steak

Prep time: 10 minutes | Cook time: 11 minutes | Serves 4

- 2½ tablespoons olive oil, divided
- 4 (4-ounce) top sirloin steaks, each 1 inch thick
- ½ teaspoon freshly ground black pepper, plus more as needed
- ½ teaspoon sea salt, plus more as needed
- 1 sprig fresh rosemary
- 1 sprig fresh thyme
- 2 garlic cloves, minced
- 1 tablespoon butter
- 1 pound green beans, trimmed

1. Heat 1½ tablespoons of olive oil in a large nonstick skillet over medium-high heat. Season the steaks with the pepper and salt. Add the rosemary, thyme, and garlic to the skillet. Add the steak and cook until browned, 3 to 4 minutes on each side.
2. Add the butter and continue to cook the steak, basting the steak with the butter constantly, for 1 to 2 minutes. Remove the skillet from the heat.
3. Bring a large pot of water to a boil over high heat. Add the green beans and cook until tender, 4 to 5 minutes.
4. Drain and toss the green beans with the remaining 1 tablespoon of olive oil and season with the salt and pepper to taste.

PER SERVING

Calories: 352 | Fat: 24 g | Protein: 26 g | Sodium: 323 mg | Fiber: 3 g | Carbohydrates: 8 g | Sugar: 2

Mushroom and Cheddar Cheeseburgers

Prep time: 10 minutes | Cook time: 5 minutes | Serves 4

- 1 large egg, beaten
- ½ cup shredded low-fat cheddar cheese
- ⅓ cup diced mushrooms
- ¼ cup finely chopped scallions
- 1 tablespoon chopped fresh cilantro
- 1 teaspoon Worcestershire sauce
- ½ teaspoon sea salt
- ¼ teaspoon freshly ground black pepper
- 1 tablespoon olive oil
- 4 100% whole wheat burger buns

1. In a large bowl, mix the ground beef, egg, cheese, mushrooms, scallions, cilantro, Worcestershire sauce, salt, and pepper. Using your hands, shape the mixture into 4 equal patties.
2. Heat the olive oil in a large nonstick skillet over medium-high heat. Add the patties and cook until cooked through, 4 to 5 minutes on each side.
3. Place each patty on a bun and add your desired toppings.

PER SERVING

Calories: 321 | Fat: 14 g | Protein: 28 g | Sodium: 629 mg | Fiber: 2 g | Carbohydrates: 20 g | Sugar: 3 g

Cheese, Tomato, and Beef Stuffed Peppers

Prep time: 15 minutes | Cook time: 29 minutes | Serves 4

- ½ cup quinoa
- 1 tablespoon olive oil
- 2 scallions, both green and white parts, finely chopped
- 3 garlic cloves, minced
- 8 ounces extra-lean ground beef
- 2 teaspoons minced fresh basil
- ½ teaspoon sea salt
- ¼ teaspoon freshly ground black pepper
- ½ cup reduced-sodium tomato sauce
- 4 red bell peppers, tops removed and seeded
- ½ cup shredded reduced-fat mozzarella cheese

1. Cook the quinoa according to the package instructions.
2. Preheat the oven to 350°F (180°C). Have a shallow baking dish ready.
3. Heat the olive oil in a large nonstick skillet over medium-high heat. Add the scallions and garlic and sauté for 1 minute. Add the ground beef and cook, breaking it apart using a wooden spoon, until it is browned and cooked through, 6 to 8 minutes.
4. Add the basil, salt, pepper, and tomato sauce and stir until combined. Remove from the heat, add the quinoa, and stir until combined.
5. Stand the peppers in the baking dish and stuff each one with equal amounts of beef and quinoa mixture. Cover the baking dish with aluminum foil and bake for 10 to 15 minutes, or until the peppers are tender. Sprinkle the cheese over the top and bake for an additional 5 minutes, or until the cheese is melted.

PER SERVING

Calories: 262 | Fat: 10 g | Protein: 20 g | Sodium: 369 mg | Fiber: 5 g | Carbohydrates: 24 g | Sugar: 2 g

Oriental Beef Muscle Stir-Fry

Prep time: 5 minutes | Cook time: 15 minutes| Serves 4

- 18oz of diced beef rump
- 1 tsp Chinese five-spice powder
- 2 cup of egg noodles
- 1 large chopped red chilli
- 1 chopped garlic clove
- 1 chopped thumb-size piece of ginger
- 1 stick lemongrass
- 2 tbsp of olive oil
- 4oz sugar snap peas
- 8 baby corns, sliced diagonally
- 6 chopped spring onions
- ½ lime
- 2 tbsp soy sauce
- 1 tbsp fish sauce
- 2 tbsp roasted peanuts
- Handful of chopped coriander, to serve

1. Get a bowl and add the beef and five-spice and leave to marinade. Place the egg noodles in a pot of boiling water for about 5 minutes, drain and then place to one side.
2. Mix together the chopped chilli, ginger, garlic and lemongrass in a bowl.
3. Add 1 tbsp of olive oil to a wok and heat on a medium heat. Add the ginger mixture into the wok and fry for 1 minute. Turn up the heat and add 1 more tbsp of olive oil to the wok and add the beef and fry until browned.
4. Add the sugar snaps, spring onions and baby corn to the wok and continue to stir-fry for around a minute before adding the egg noodles and mix together. Turn off the heat and add the soy sauce, fish sauces and squeezed lime juice.
5. Place in a bowl and add the peanuts and chopped coriander to serve.

PER SERVING

Calories: 349 | protein: 34g|carbs: 26g|fat: 14g

Bulk-Up Lamb Curry and Peanut Stew

Prep time: 5 minutes | Cook time: 2 hours 5 minutes| Serves 4

- 1/2 cup chopped peanuts
- 1/2 cup canned coconut cream
- 4 tbsp massaman curry paste
- 24oz diced lamb steak (or beef)
- 16oz chopped white potatoes
- 1 chopped onion
- 1 cinnamon stick
- 1 tbsp tamarind paste
- 1 tbsp fish sauce
- 1 sliced red chilli

1. Pre-heat oven (375°F/190 °C/Gas Mark 5).
2. Get a large casserole dish and place on the gas/ electric hob on a medium heat.
3. Add 2 tbsp of coconut cream and the curry paste and fry for around a minute before adding the diced lamb. Stir in and brown. Add the rest of the coconut cream with a cup of water as well as the potatoes, onions, cinnamon stick, tamarind, fish sauce and peanuts.
4. Reduce heat to a simmer, cover the casserole, transfer to the oven and cook for 2 hours until the lamb is soft and tender.
5. Add the sliced chilli to the top and serve.

PER SERVING

Calories: 600 | protein: 44g|carbs: 38g|fat: 46g

Steak and Cheese Muscle Club

Prep time: 5 minutes | Cook time: 15 minutes| Serves 4

- 18oz of diced beef rump
- 1 tsp Chinese five-spice powder
- 2 cup of egg noodles
- 1 large chopped red chilli
- 1 chopped garlic clove
- 1 chopped thumb-size piece of ginger
- 1 stick lemongrass
- 2 tbsp of olive oil
- 4oz sugar snap peas
- 8 baby corns, sliced diagonally
- 2 tbsp soy sauce
- 1 tbsp fish sauce
- 2 tbsp roasted peanuts
- Handful of chopped coriander, to serve

1. Heat up a griddle pan on a high heat until very hot. Drizzle the olive oil over both sides of the steak. Sprinkle some salt and pepper over it and place the steak in the pan and fry for 3 minutes on each side. Place the steak to one side and leave to rest for a minute.
2. Cut in half to form two slices of steak.
3. Cut the whole-wheat rolls in half and place toast. Once done, add the mustard and rocket to the roll and place 1 half of the steak on top. Add balsamic vinegar and the cheese to the top and then make the sandwich.
4. Repeat steps with the other roll.

PER SERVING

Calories: 332 | protein: 32g|carbs: 27g|fat: 11g

Anabolic Pork Soup

Prep time: 5 minutes | Cook time: 25 minutes| Serves 4

- 16oz diced pork steaks
- 1 cup chicken stock
- 1 tbsp soy sauce
- 2 tsp Chinese five-spice powder
- 1 piece ginger finely chopped
- 1 cup of baby spinach
- 1 tsp of chopped red chilli,
- 1.5 cup of rice noodles
- Handful of chopped spring onions

1. Get a large saucepan and add all the ingredients except for the spring onions and noodles. Cover the pan and bring to a simmer on a medium heat.
2. Without letting the ingredients boil, leave to cook for around 8-10 minutes.
3. While cooking the pork, place the rice noodles in a pot of boiling water for about 5 minutes and then drain.
4. Drain and place the noodles in a bowl and add the pork and greens over the noodles. Sprinkle the spring onions over the dish and serve.

PER SERVING

Calories: 297 | protein: 21g|carbs: 13g|fat: 17g

Super Steak with Spicy Rice and Beans

Prep time: 5 minutes | Cook time: 45 minutes| Serves 2

- 2 12oz sirloin steaks
- 4 tsp olive oil
- 1 small onion, sliced
- 1 cup brown long-grain rice
- 1½tsp fajita seasoning
- 1 can of drained kidney beans
- Handful of chopped coriander leaves
- 2 tbsp tomato salsa, to serve

1. Pour 3 tsp of oil into a deep saucepan on a medium heat and add the onion. Fry the onion for around 4 minutes.
2. Then add ½ the fajita seasoning and long grain rice. Cook for 1 minute. Add 300ml of boiling water to the saucepan and stir in. Cover the saucepan and let simmer for 20 minutes until the water has been absorbed and the rice is fluffy. Add the kidney beans and keep the pan warm.
3. While the rice is cooking, sprinkle salt and pepper over the steak as well as ½ fajita seasoning. Pre-heat a griddle pan on a high heat, add the steaks and cook for 8 minutes in total, turning the steaks half way through.
4. Add the rice to a bowl and mix in the coriander. Add a tbsp of tomato salsa to each of the steaks and serve.

PER SERVING

Calories: 650 | protein: 48g|carbs: 60g|fat: 26g

Muscle Mint Lamb Steaks

Prep time: 5 minutes | Cook time: 45 minutes| Serves 4

- 4 8oz lamb leg steaks
- 2 tbsp olive oil
- 2 chopped garlic cloves
- 1 tbsp balsamic vinegar
- Handful of chopped mint leaves

1. Get a bowl and add the mint, vinegar and garlic and mix together.
2. Add the lamb to the bowl and leave to marinade for at least 30 minutes.
3. Pre-heat a griddle pan on a medium to high heat and cook the lamb for 4 minutes each side or until cooked through.
4. Serve alone or with your choice of salad for a delicious accompaniment.

PER SERVING

Calories: 367 | protein: 41g|carbs: 2g|fat: 22g

Mighty Lamb Casserole

Prep time: 5 minutes | Cook time: 2 hours| Serves 2

- 18oz of diced beef rump
- 1 tsp Chinese five-spice powder
- 2 cup of egg noodles
- 1 large chopped red chilli
- 1 chopped garlic clove
- 1 chopped thumb-size piece of ginger
- 1 stick lemongrass
- 2 tbsp of olive oil
- 4oz sugar snap peas
- 8 baby corns, sliced diagonally
- 6 chopped spring onions
- ½ lime
- 2 tbsp soy sauce
- 1 tbsp fish sauce
- 2 tbsp roasted peanuts
- Handful of chopped coriander, to serve

1. Get a large casserole dish and heat the olive oil on a medium heat.
2. Add the lamb to the casserole dish and cook for 5 minutes until browned, then add the chopped onion and carrots. Leave to cook for another 5 minutes until the vegetables begin to soften.
3. Add the chicken stock, kale and rosemary. Then cover the casserole, leave to simmer on a low heat for 1-1.5 hours until the lamb is tender and fully cooked through.
4. Add the cannellini beans 15 minutes before the end of the cooking time.
5. Plate up and serve with the chopped parsley to garnish.

PER SERVING

Calories: 380 | protein: 35g|carbs: 33g|fat: 9g

Farley'S Muscle Building Chilli Con Carne

Prep time: 5 minutes | Cook time: 1 hour 25 minutes| Serves 4

- 20oz lean ground beef
- 1 tbsp oil
- 1 chopped onion
- 1 chopped red pepper
- 2 crushed garlic cloves,
- 1 tsp of chilli powder
- 1 tsp paprika
- 1 tsp ground cumin
- 1 beef stock cube
- 16oz of tinned chopped tomatoes
- 2 tbsp tomato purée
- 16oz of dried and rinsed red kidney beans
- 1 cup of brown rice

1. Get a pan and add the olive oil and heat on a medium heat.
2. Add the onions to the pan and fry until soft.
3. Then add the garlic, red pepper, chilli powder, paprika and cumin. Stir together and cook for 5 minutes.
4. Add the ground mince to the pan and cook until browned.
5. Get 300ml of hot water and add the beef stock cube to it. Add this to the pan along with the chopped tomatoes. Also add the puree and stir in well. Bring the pan to a simmer, cover and cook for around 50 minutes. Stir occasionally.
6. After 30 minutes and while the mince is cooking, add 300ml of cold water to a separate pot and heat until the water is boiling. Once boiling, add the rice and leave for 20 minutes.
7. Once the rice is done, drain and put to one side. Add the beans to the meat mix and cook for another 10 minutes.
8. Serve the rice topped with the chilli con carne.

PER SERVING

Calories: 389 | protein: 37g|carbs: 25g|fat: 17g

Super Lamb Steaks with Mediterranean Veg

Prep time: 5 minutes | Cook time: 10 minutes| Serves 4

- 2 8oz lamb breast steaks
- 2 chopped courgettes
- 2 tbsp olive oil
- Handful of rocket
- 2 garlic cloves, chopped
- 8 halved baby cherry tomatoes
- Handful of chopped coriander

1. Preheat the grill.
2. Add the oil to a pan and heat on a medium heat.
3. Throw in the courgettes, tomatoes and garlic and fry until courgettes and tomatoes are soft.
4. Add the rocket and coriander and stir in.
5. Meanwhile, sprinkle some salt and pepper over the lamb steaks. Place the lamb on a tray and grill for 4 minutes. each side.
6. Serve alongside the veg.

PER SERVING

Calories: 308 | protein: 34g|carbs: 15g|fat: 14g

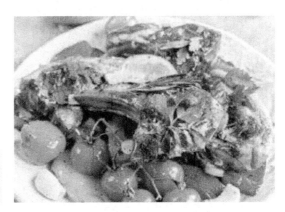

Mass Gaining Lamb Flatbread

Prep time: 5 minutes | Cook time: 15 minutes| Serves 4

- 2 8oz lamb leg steaks
- 1 tbsp harissa
- 4 whole meal flatbreads
- 4 tbsp of organic houmous
- Handful of baby spinach
- Handful of watercress
- A pinch of salt and pepper

1. Preheat the grill.
2. Sprinkle harissa, salt and pepper over the lamb.
3. Place lamb on a baking tray and grill for 4 minutes before turning the lamb over and cooking for a further 4 minutes. Take the tray out of the grill and leave to one side.
4. Place the flatbreads under the grill for around 1 – 2 minutes before removing and spreading on the houmous.
5. Cut the lamb into thin strips and place over the flat bread.
6. Add the baby spinach and watercress, roll the flatbread into a wrap and enjoy.

PER SERVING

Calories: 391 | protein: 29g|carbs: 34g|fat: 17g

Muscle Building Steak and Sweet Potato Fries

Prep time: 5 minutes | Cook time: 35 minutes| Serves 4

- 4oz of sirloin steak
- 8oz of sweet potatoes cut into chips
- 1 tbsp olive oil
- 1 chopped red onion
- 1 bag of pre-washed salad
- 1 tbsp of balsamic vinegar
- A pinch of black pepper

1. Pre-Heat oven (375°F/190 °C/Gas Mark 5).
2. Get a baking tray, spread the chips out and bake for around 25 minutes.
3. While the chips are cooking, get a large frying pan and heat the olive oil on a medium heat.
4. Pepper the steaks and add to the pan. Fry the steaks for 6 minutes in total, turning the steaks once halfway through.
5. Take the steak and leave to cool.
6. Get a large bowl and add the salad and chopped onion. Drizzle with the vinegar and serve with the potatoes and steak.
7. the cheese and pine nuts and let the cheese melt for a further 4-5 minutes.
8. Plate up and serve.

PER SERVING

Calories: 418 | protein: 29g|carbs: 39g|fat: 15g

Strength and Mass Meatloaf

Prep time: 5 minutes | Cook time: 55 minutes| Serves 4

- 36oz of lean ground beef
- 1 tsp olive oil
- 1 chopped red onion
- 1 tsp garlic
- 3 chopped tomatoes
- 1 whole beaten egg
- 1cup of whole wheat bread crumbs
- Handful of parsley
- 1/4 cup of low fat parmesan
- 1/2 cup of organic skim milk
- A pinch of salt and pepper
- 1 tsp oregano

1. Preheat the oven to (400°F/200 °C/Gas Mark 6).
2. Add the oil to a pan and heat on a medium heat.
3. Cook the onions until soft but not browned. Remove the onions from the pan and let cool.
4. Get a big bowl and mix all of the ingredients together.
5. Put the meat in a big baking tray and cook on a high heat for around 30-35 minutes.
6. Serve once cooked through and piping hot.

PER SERVING

Calories: 410 | protein: 47g|carbs: 15g|fat: 19g

Tasty Beef Broccoli Stir Fry

Prep time: 5 minutes | Cook time: 15 minutes| Serves 4

- 16oz of diced frying beef steaks
- 1 head of broccoli, broken into florets
- 4 chopped celery sticks
- Handful of sweet corn
- 1 cup beef stock
- 2 tbsp of horseradish sauce
- 1 tbsp of olive oil
- A pinch of salt and pepper

1. Heat the olive oil on a medium/high heat in a frying pan.
2. Add some salt and pepper to the beefsteaks and place in the frying pan.
3. Stir-fry for 2 minutes until the beef is browned then remove and set aside.
4. Add the broccoli and chopped celery to the pan and fry for a further 2 minutes.
5. Add the beef stock to the pan, then cover. Reduce the heat and let the veg simmer for 2 minutes.
6. Place the steak back in the pan and mix with the other vegetables for another minute.
7. Plate up and serve with the horseradish sauce.

PER SERVING

Calories: 277 | protein: 30g|carbs: 7g|fat: 14g

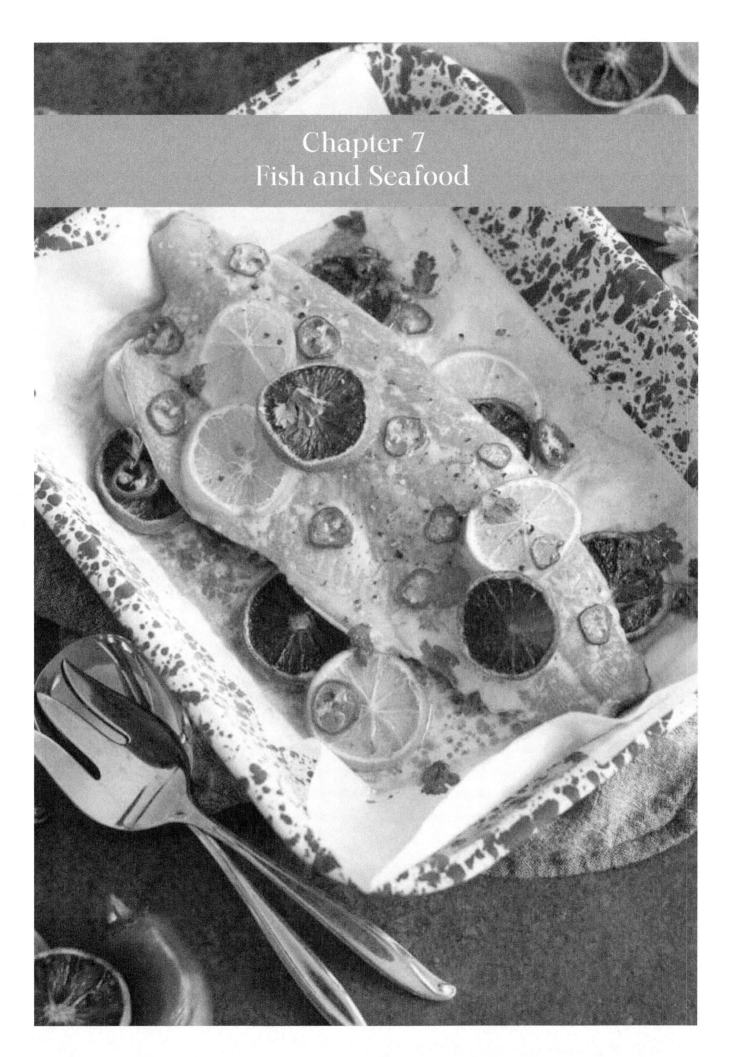

Chapter 7
Fish and Seafood

Shrimp Creole

Prep time: 10| Cook time: 1 hour| Makes 4 (4-ounce) servings

- 1 tablespoon extra-virgin olive oil
- ½ cup (1 stalk) celery, chopped
- ½ cup (about 1 medium) onion, chopped
- ½ teaspoon minced garlic
- 1 (16-ounce) can petite diced tomatoes
- 1 (8-ounce) can tomato sauce
- 1 teaspoon soy sauce (gluten-free, if desired) or liquid aminos
- 1 teaspoon apple cider vinegar
- ¼ teaspoon freshly squeezed lemon juice
- 1½ teaspoons granulated stevia or honey
- 1½ teaspoons salt
- ½ teaspoon chili powder
- 2 teaspoons corn starch
- 2 teaspoons water
- ½ cup (1 medium) green bell pepper, diced
- 1 pound jumbo shrimp, peeled and deveined

1. In a large skillet over medium-high heat, heat the olive oil. Add the celery, onion, and garlic, and cook until tender, but not brown, about 5 minutes.
2. Add the tomatoes, tomato sauce, soy sauce, apple cider vinegar, lemon juice, stevia, salt, and chili powder. Simmer uncovered for at least 20 minutes, and up to 45 minutes, stirring occasionally.
3. In a small bowl, mix the cornstarch and water. Stir the mixture into the skillet, and cook until the sauce is thick and bubbly.
4. Add the bell pepper and shrimp, cover, and simmer for 5 minutes more.
5. Divide among four bowls and enjoy.

PER SERVING

Calories: 168 |carbs: 11.8g|fat: 3g|protein 22.3g

Coconut Shrimp with Sweet and Spicy Dipping Sauce

Prep time: 20 minutes| Cook time: 15 minutes| Serves 6

FOR THE SHRIMP

- 3 tablespoons corn starch
- 3 egg whites
- 6 tablespoons shredded coconut, unsweetened
- 2 tablespoons granulated stevia
- 24 medium shrimp, peeled, deveined, and tails on
- FOR THE DIPPING SAUCE
- ¼ cup sugar-free orange marmalade
- 1 teaspoon sriracha

TO MAKE THE SHRIMP

1. Preheat the oven to 375°F.
2. Line a baking sheet with parchment paper.
3. Put the cornstarch in a small bowl.
4. In a second small bowl, whip the egg whites until stiff peaks form.
5. In a third small bowl, mix the coconut and stevia.
6. Set the three bowls in a row. Take one shrimp by

the tail, coat it in cornstarch, and then dip it in the whipped egg whites, the more volume the better. Finally, coat the shrimp in the coconut, and place it on the baking sheet.

7. Bake at 375°F for 10 to 15 minutes, turning over after about 7 minutes. The shrimp are done when the coconut has toasted and the tails are pink. (The egg white, if exposed, will still be white.)

TO MAKE THE DIPPING SAUCE

8. While the shrimp are in the oven, in a small bowl, mix the marmalade with the sriracha. If necessary, add a little water, 1 teaspoon at a time, to thin out the dipping sauce as needed.
9. Serve the shrimp warm with the dipping sauce.

PER SERVING

Calories: 168 |carbs: 8.7g|fat: 3.5g|protein 22.2g

Cioppino

Prep time: 30 mins| Cook time: 50 mins| Serves 8

- 1 tablespoon extra-virgin olive oil
- 1 large fennel bulb, thinly sliced
- 1 large white onion, chopped
- 3 large shallots, chopped
- 1 teaspoon salt (optional), plus more if desired
- 2 teaspoons minced garlic
- 1 teaspoon red pepper flakes, plus more if desired
- ¼ cup tomato paste
- ¾ cup water
- 1 dried bay leaf
- 1 pound Manila clams, scrubbed
- 1 pound mussels, scrubbed and debearded
- 1 pound large shrimp, peeled and deveined
- 1½ pounds mahimahi fillets, cut into 2-inch chunks

1. In a large soup pot over medium heat, heat the olive oil. Add the fennel, onion, shallots, and salt (if using), and cook for 10 minutes, stirring frequently, until the onion is translucent.
2. Add the garlic and red pepper flakes, and cook for 2 minutes more.
3. Stir in the tomato paste, tomatoes with their juices, fish stock, lemon juice, water, and bay leaf. Cover and bring to a simmer, and then reduce the heat to medium-low. Continue to simmer for 30 minutes.
4. Add the clams and mussels, cover, and cook for about 5 minutes, until the clams and mussels begin to open.
5. Add the shrimp and fish, and cook for about 5 minutes more, until the fish and shrimp are cooked through and the clams and mussels are completely open. Stir gently, careful not to break apart the fish.
6. Discard the bay leaf and any clams and mussels that failed to open.
7. Ladle a little of each shellfish, a little mahimahi, and some soup into each bowl, season with more salt and red pepper flakes as desired, and serve.

PER SERVING

Calories: 226 |carbs: 11.8g|fat: 5.1g|protein 31.3g

Scallop Stir-Fry

Prep time: 15 minutes| Cook time: 10 minutes| Serves 4

FOR THE MARINADE

- 2 tablespoons soy sauce, (gluten-free, if desired) or liquid aminos
- 2 tablespoons freshly squeezed lemon juice
- ¼ cup rice vinegar
- 2 tablespoons honey
- 1 tablespoon corn starch
- 2 teaspoons apple cider vinegar
- 1 garlic clove, crushed
- Pinch freshly ground black pepper

FOR THE SCALLOPS

- 1 pound large scallops
- 1 teaspoon peanut oil or coconut oil
- 1 pound small baby bok choy, ends trimmed
- 1 pound white mushrooms, sliced
- 1 pound fresh snow peas
- 1 red bell pepper, cut into ½-inch pieces
- 1 onion, quartered, layers separated

TO MAKE THE MARINADE

1. In a small bowl, mix well to combine the soy sauce, lemon juice, rice vinegar, honey, cornstarch, apple cider vinegar, garlic, and pepper.

TO MAKE THE SCALLOPS

2. Pat the scallops dry with paper towels. In a medium bowl, drizzle the scallops with less than half of the marinade. Toss to coat.
3. Heat a large skillet over medium-high heat. Add the oil, and swirl to coat the pan. Add the scallops, and sear for 1 minute on each side. Remove and set aside.
4. Add the bok choy, mushrooms, snow peas, bell peppers, and onion to the skillet, and cook for about 5 minutes, until tender. Add the remaining marinade, and cook until heated through. Add the scallops back into the skillet, and cook for 1 more minute.
5. Divide among four plates and serve.

PER SERVING

Calories: 171 |carbs: 22g|fat: 2.8g|protein 15.8g

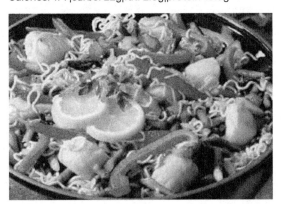

Maple and Mustard Baked Scallops

Prep time: 5 minutes| Cook time: 30 minutes| Serves 1

- 4 jumbo sea scallops (about 4 ounces)
- 1½ teaspoons Dijon mustard
- 1½ teaspoons real maple syrup

1. Preheat the oven to 350°F.
2. Place the scallops on a foil-lined baking sheet 1½ inches apart.
3. In a small bowl, mix the mustard and maple syrup. Spoon the mixture evenly over the scallops, and spread to coat the top.
4. Bake for 20 to 30 minutes, depending on size, until opaque.
5. Enjoy warm.

PER SERVING

Calories: 125|carbs: 10g|fat: 1g|protein :17g

Tuna Melt Stuffed Tomatoes

Prep time: 15 minutes| Cook time: 5 minutes| Serves 2

- 1 (7-ounce) can tuna in water, drained
- 2 tablespoons nonfat Greek yogurt
- 1 tablespoon chopped fresh basil
- 1 tablespoon diced red bell pepper
- 1 tablespoon diced red onion
- Pinch freshly ground black pepper
- 2 large tomatoes
- ¼ cup shredded low-fat mozzarella, divided
- 2 pinches crushed red pepper, divided

1. Preheat the broiler to high. In a small bowl, use a fork to mix the tuna, yogurt, basil, bell pepper, onion, and black pepper until well blended.
2. Slice off the top of each tomato with a sharp knife, and use a spoon to hollow out the tomatoes.
3. Stuff the tuna mixture into the tomato cups, and press down firmly with a fork.
4. Place the stuffed tomatoes in a loaf pan or baking dish. Top each with 2 tablespoons of shredded mozzarella and a pinch of crushed red pepper.
5. Broil 6 to 8 inches from the heat for 3 to 5 minutes, until the cheese melts and slightly browns.
6. Serve immediately. The stuffed tomatoes go well with salad greens or a veggie side dish.

PER SERVING

Calories: 189 |carbs: 10g|fat: 3.9g|protein: 31g

Almond-Crusted Baked Cod

Prep time: 15 minutes| Cook time: 15 minutes| Serves 4

- 1 large egg
- 2 egg whites
- ½ cup blanched almond flour
- ½ teaspoon mustard powder
- ¼ teaspoon ground cayenne pepper
- ¼ teaspoon garlic powder
- 4 (6-ounce) cod fillets
- Extra-virgin olive oil spray

1. Preheat the oven to 350°F.
2. Line a baking sheet with nonstick aluminum foil or a silicone baking mat.
3. In a medium bowl, whisk the egg and egg whites. Set aside.
4. In a large bowl, mix together the almond flour, mustard, cayenne pepper, and garlic powder.
5. On a work surface, pat the cod dry with paper towels. Dip a cod fillet into the egg, coating both sides. Shake off any excess. Dredge in the almond flour mixture, coating both sides, and place the seasoned cod on the prepared baking sheet. Repeat with the remaining cod.
6. Lightly spray each breaded fillet with olive oil spray. Bake for 15 minutes.
7. Plate the fish and serve fresh from the oven.

PER SERVING

Calories: 245 |carbs: 3g|fat: 9.5g|protein: 36.5g

Salmon-Quinoa Cakes

Prep time: 15 minutes| Cook time: 30 minutes| Serves 6

- 1 (7-ounce) can Alaskan salmon, undrained
- 1½ cups cooked quinoa
- ½ cup shredded (1 medium beet or 1½ medium carrots)
- ¼ cup finely diced onion, any color
- 1½ teaspoons minced garlic
- ½ teaspoon dried parsley or ¼ cup chopped fresh parsley
- 1 egg
- 2 egg whites
- ¼ cup nonfat Greek yogurt
- ¼ cup nutritional yeast
- ½ teaspoon salt
- 1 teaspoon coconut oil or extra-virgin olive oil

1. In a large bowl, stir together the salmon and its liquid with the quinoa. Add the beet, onion, garlic, and parsley, and mix well.
2. In a medium bowl, use a fork to beat the egg, egg whites, yogurt, nutritional yeast, and salt together.
3. Add the egg mixture to the salmon and quinoa mixture, and stir until well combined.
4. Heat a large skillet over medium heat. Add the oil, and swirl to coat.
5. Using a ¼-cup measuring cup, scoop as many cakes into the skillet as will fit without the edges touching. Do not overcrowd. Fry for 5 to 8 minutes, until the bottoms brown and the cakes are firm. Flip and brown the other side, 3 to 5 minutes more.
6. Transfer to a dish to keep warm, and continue frying until all of the mixture has been used. The batter should make close to 18 cakes.
7. Serve warm.

PER SERVING

Calories: 160 |carbs: 14.5g|fat: 5.9g|protein :13g

Coconut-Seared Scallops with Wilted Spinach

Prep time: 5 minutes| Cook time: 10 minutes| Serves 1

FOR THE WILTED SPINACH

- 1½ teaspoons coconut oil
- 1 (10-ounce) bag baby spinach
- Pinch freshly grated nutmeg

FOR THE SEARED SCALLOPS

- 1½ teaspoons coconut oil
- 4 jumbo sea scallops (about 4 ounces)
- Salt

TO MAKE THE SPINACH

1. Heat a skillet over medium-high heat. Add the coconut oil, and swirl the skillet to coat the bottom.
2. Fill the skillet with spinach leaves. Cook, stirring, until wilted, about a minute. Add more spinach to the skillet, and repeat the process until all of the spinach is wilted.
3. Transfer the spinach to a plate, and lightly dust with nutmeg.

TO MAKE THE SCALLOPS

4. Return the skillet to medium-high heat, add the coconut oil, and swirl to coat the bottom.
5. On a work surface, pat the scallops dry with paper towels, season with salt, and add to the skillet. Cook undisturbed for 1 to 2 minutes, until the bottoms brown. Flip, season with salt, and cook for another 1 to 2 minutes. They will be browned on both sides and cooked through but still slightly pink in the center.
6. Place the scallops atop the wilted spinach and enjoy.

PER SERVING

Calories: 277 |carbs: 12g|fat:16g|protein 25g

Bourbon Lime Salmon

Prep time: 5 minutes | Cook time: 15 minutes| Serves 8

- 1 cup packed brown sugar
- 6 tablespoons bourbon
- ¼ cup low-sodium soy sauce or coconut aminos
- 2 tablespoons lime juice
- 2 teaspoons grated fresh ginger
- ½ teaspoon salt
- ¼ teaspoon ground black pepper
- 2 cloves garlic, peeled and crushed
- 8 (6-ounce) salmon fillets
- 4 teaspoons sesame seeds
- ½ cup sliced scallions

1. Combine brown sugar, bourbon, soy sauce, lime juice, ginger, salt, pepper, and garlic in a large re-sealable plastic bag. Marinate salmon fillets in the bag at least 30 minutes in the refrigerator.
2. Preheat broiler.
3. Transfer fish to a broiler pan and discard marinade. Broil fish 10–12 minutes until it flakes easily.
4. Sprinkle fish with sesame seeds and scallions and serve.

PER SERVING

Calories:476 | Fat: 20g | Sodium: 255mg|
Carbohydrates:27g | Fiber: 0g| Sugar: 0g | Protein: 44g

Healthy Fish and Chips

Prep time: 5 minutes | Cook time: 35 minutes| Serves 4

- 1 medium sweet potato, peeled and cut crosswise into ⅛" slices
- 1 medium russet potato, cut crosswise into ⅛" slices
- 2 tablespoons olive oil, divided
- ¼ teaspoon dried rosemary
- 1 teaspoon salt, divided
- ½ teaspoon ground black pepper, divided
- 1 large egg white, beaten
- 2 tablespoons unsweetened almond milk
- ¼ cup almond flour
- ¼ cup dried bread crumbs
- 4 (4-ounce) cod fillets

1. Preheat oven to 450°F. Line a large baking sheet with parchment paper. Spray a 9" × 9" baking pan lightly with nonstick cooking spray.
2. In a large bowl, toss sweet potato, potato, 1 tablespoon oil, rosemary, ½ teaspoon salt, and ¼ teaspoon pepper.
3. Arrange slices in a single layer on the prepared baking sheet. Bake for 18–20 minutes until browned and crisp, tossing at the halfway mark.
4. Meanwhile, combine egg white and almond milk in a shallow bowl. In another shallow bowl, combine almond flour, bread crumbs, remaining ½ teaspoon salt, and remaining ¼ teaspoon pepper.
5. Dip each piece of fish into egg mixture, then in the bread crumb mixture. Place fillets in the pre-

pared baking dish and drizzle with the remaining 1 tablespoon oil.
6. Bake fish for 8–10 minutes until fish flakes easily when tested with a fork.
7. Serve fish with sweet potatoes and potatoes.

PER SERVING

Calories:399 | Fat: 20g | Sodium:1,072mg |
Carbohydrates: 32g| Fiber: 2g| Sugar: 0g | Protein: 23g

Grilled Tuna Teriyaki

Prep time: 5 minutes | Cook time: 55 minutes| Serves 4

- 2 tablespoons low-sodium soy sauce or coconut aminos
- 1 tablespoon rice wine vinegar
- 1 tablespoon minced fresh ginger
- 1 clove garlic, peeled and minced
- 1 tablespoon vegetable oil
- 4 (6-ounce) tuna steaks

1. In a small bowl, whisk together soy sauce, vinegar, ginger, garlic, and oil.
2. Place tuna in a shallow baking dish and pour three-quarters of the marinade over it. Set aside to marinate for 30 minutes, flipping tuna to marinate the other side after 15 minutes.
3. Preheat a gas or charcoal grill.
4. Place tuna steaks on the grill and cook for 4–5 minutes for rare or 6–8 minutes for medium-rare. Carefully flip, brush with remaining marinade, and grill another 4 minutes for rare or 5–6 minutes for medium-rare.
5. Remove from grill and serve.

PER SERVING

Calories:267 | Fat: 5g | Sodium:519mg |
Carbohydrates:1g | Fiber: 0g| Sugar:0 g | Protein: 55g

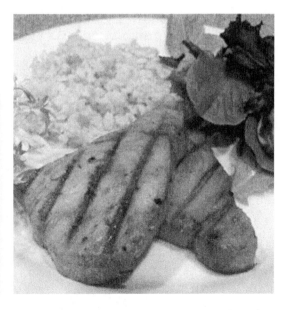

Lemon Dill Salmon

Prep time: 5 minutes | Cook time: 30 minutes| Serves 4

- 1 (1 ½-pound) salmon fillet
- 1 tablespoon salted butter or ghee, melted
- 2 teaspoons minced garlic
- 2 tablespoons chopped fresh dill
- 2 tablespoons lemon juice
- 1 tablespoon lemon zest
- ½ teaspoon salt

1. Preheat oven to 375°F.
2. Line a baking sheet with foil and center salmon on the foil.
3. In a small bowl, mix together butter, garlic, dill, lemon juice, lemon zest, and salt.
4. Pour mixture over salmon. Fold up the ends of the foil so that salmon is sealed in a pouch. Bake for 15–20 minutes until fish flakes with a fork. Serve immediately.

PER SERVING

Calories: 200| Fat: 7g | Sodium:471mg |
Carbohydrates:0g | Fiber: 0g| Sugar: 0g | Protein: 35g

Baked Coconut-Crusted Cod

Prep time: 5 minutes | Cook time: 25 minutes| Serves 2

- 2 tablespoons honey
- 1 tablespoon lime juice
- ½ cup unsweetened shredded coconut
- ½ cup panko bread crumbs
- ½ teaspoon salt
- ½ teaspoon cayenne pepper
- 2 (6-ounce) cod fillets

1. Preheat oven to 425°F. Line a baking sheet with parchment paper.
2. In a shallow bowl, combine honey and lime juice. In another shallow bowl, combine coconut, bread crumbs, salt, and pepper.
3. Dip fillets in honey mixture and then dredge in coconut and bread crumb mixture.
4. Place fillets on the prepared baking sheet and bake for 18–20 minutes until coconut turns a golden brown and fish flakes easily with a fork. Serve immediately.

PER SERVING

Calories: 439| Fat: 24g | Sodium:707mg |
Carbohydrates:37g | Fiber:6g| Sugar: 22g | Protein: 24g

Foolproof Pan-Seared Scallops

Prep time: 5 minutes | Cook time: 15 minutes| Serves 2

- ½ pound sea scallops
- ¼ teaspoon salt
- ⅛ teaspoon ground black pepper
- 3 tablespoons salted butter, divided
- 1 ½ tablespoons lemon juice
- ¼ cup dry white wine

1. Rinse scallops with water and then lay them on a paper towel. Season with salt and pepper.
2. In a large stainless steel or cast iron skillet, melt 2 tablespoons butter over medium-high heat.
3. Once the butter is melted and sizzling, place scallops into skillet.
4. Allow scallops to cook for about 5 minutes. Wait to flip them until they freely pull away from the pan.
5. Cook for another 3 minutes on the other side. Transfer scallops to a plate, drizzle with lemon juice, and keep warm.
6. Add wine to the pan with remaining 1 tablespoon butter. Cook, stirring occasionally, until reduced by half, about 3 minutes. Drizzle sauce over scallops and serve immediately.

PER SERVING

Calories: 275| Fat: 17g | Sodium: 879mg| Carbohydrates: 6g| Fiber: 0g| Sugar: 0g | Protein: 23g

Pecan-Crusted Salmon

Prep time: 5 minutes | Cook time: 18 minutes| Serves 4

- 2 tablespoons Dijon mustard
- 2 tablespoons maple syrup
- 4 (6-ounce) salmon fillets
- ½ cup finely chopped pecans

1. Preheat oven to 425°F. Spray a 9" × 13" baking dish with nonstick cooking spray.
2. In a small bowl, mix together mustard and maple syrup.
3. Place fillets in a single layer in the prepared baking dish. Spread mustard mixture over fillets. Sprinkle with pecans, pressing them into the mustard mixture.
4. Bake for 12–15 minutes until salmon is cooked through and flakes easily with a fork. Serve immediately.

PER SERVING

Calories: 446| Fat: 25g | Sodium:276mg |
Carbohydrates:9g | Fiber: 2g| Sugar: 7g | Protein: 45g

Maple Mustard Tuna Steaks

Prep time: 5 minutes | Cook time: 25 minutes| Serves 4

- 3 tablespoons maple syrup
- 1 ½ tablespoons Dijon mustard
- 1 ½ tablespoons lemon juice
- 2 teaspoons extra-virgin olive oil
- 4 (5-ounce, 1"-thick) tuna steaks
- ½ teaspoon salt
- ¼ teaspoon ground black pepper

1. In a shallow bowl, combine maple syrup, mustard, lemon juice, and oil. Reserve 2 tablespoons of maple and mustard mixture and set aside.
2. Add tuna to remaining maple and mustard mixture and turn to coat. Set aside to marinate for 10 minutes, turning once after 5 minutes.
3. Coat a large stainless steel or cast iron skillet with nonstick cooking spray and heat over medium-high heat.
4. Remove tuna from marinade and season with salt and pepper.
5. Place tuna in pan and cook for 1–2 minutes on each side until lightly seared on the outside.
6. Remove tuna from pan. Drizzle with reserved maple and mustard mixture and serve.

PER SERVING

Calories:218 | Fat: 4g | Sodium: 347mg| Carbohydrates: 10g| Fiber: 0g| Sugar: 9g | Protein: 35g

Cod with Bacon, Red Onion, and Kale

Prep time: 5 minutes | Cook time: 25 minutes| Serves 2

- 4 slices thick-cut bacon, chopped
- 2 (6-ounce) cod fillets
- 1 medium red onion, peeled and sliced
- 4 cups roughly chopped kale leaves
- ¼ teaspoon salt

1. In a large skillet, cook bacon for 5–7 minutes over medium-high heat until slightly crisp. Remove bacon and set aside, leaving the remaining fat in the pan.
2. Add fillets to the pan and sear for 4 minutes, then remove and set aside. (Fillets won't be fully cooked at this point.)
3. Add onion to the pan and sauté for 2 minutes. Add kale and salt. Sauté for another 1–2 minutes until onion is soft and kale begins to wilt.
4. Return fillets to the skillet and cover with a lid. Cook for 7–8 minutes until cod flakes easily with a fork.
5. Divide cod, onion, and kale between two plates. Top with bacon and serve immediately.

PER SERVING

Calories:358 | Fat: 18g | Sodium:1,156mg | Carbohydrates: 20g| Fiber: 2g| Sugar: 5g | Protein: 30g

Tuna Salad Plate

Prep time: 5 minutes | Cook time: 5 minutes| Serves 1

- 1 (5-ounce) can solid white tuna, drained
- 1 teaspoon mayonnaise
- 2 teaspoons sweet relish
- 1 large hard-cooked egg, peeled and sliced
- ½ medium avocado, peeled, pitted, and sliced
- ½ medium cucumber, sliced
- ¼ teaspoon salt
- ⅛ teaspoon ground black pepper

1. In a small bowl, combine tuna, mayonnaise, and sweet relish. Place tuna mixture on a plate.
2. Arrange egg, avocado, and cucumber slices around tuna mixture. Season with salt and pepper and serve.

PER SERVING

Calories: 307| Fat: 16g | Sodium:1,122mg | Carbohydrates: 5g| Fiber: 3g| Sugar: 0g | Protein: 40g

Homemade Fish Sticks

Prep time: 5 minutes | Cook time: 10 minutes| Serves 4

- 1 ½ cups dried bread crumbs
- ½ cup grated Parmesan cheese
- ½ tablespoon onion salt
- ¼ teaspoon salt
- ⅓ cup almond flour
- 1 large egg
- 1 tablespoon water
- 2 (6-ounce) flounder fillets
- 2 tablespoons olive oil

1. In a shallow bowl, combine bread crumbs, cheese, onion salt, and salt. Place almond flour in a second shallow bowl. In a third shallow bowl, whisk egg with water.
2. Remove skin and cut fillets into eight strips of equal size.
3. Dust fish with almond flour, then dip in egg mixture. Finally, dredge fish in the bread crumb mixture.
4. Heat oil in a large skillet. In two batches, fry fish for 2 minutes per side until golden brown. Serve hot.

PER SERVING

Calories: 331| Fat:16 g | Sodium: 1,180mg| Carbohydrates: 25g| Fiber:1 g| Sugar: 0g | Protein: 22g

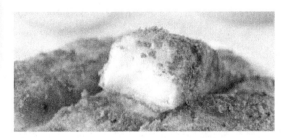

Garlic and Herb Seared Salmon

Prep time: 5 minutes | Cook time: 15 minutes| Serves 4

- 4 teaspoons minced garlic
- 1 teaspoon dried herbes de Provence
- 1 teaspoon red wine vinegar
- 1 teaspoon plus 2 tablespoons olive oil, divided
- 2 tablespoons Dijon mustard
- 4 (6-ounce) wild-caught salmon fillets
- 4 lemon wedges

1. Combine garlic, herbs, vinegar, 1 teaspoon oil, and mustard in a small bowl. Set aside.
2. Heat remaining 2 tablespoons oil in a large nonstick skillet over medium-high heat. Add salmon and cook 5 minutes.
3. Flip fillets and cook 3 minutes, spooning half the garlic sauce on the cooked side of each fillet.
4. Flip fillets again, cooking 1 more minute and spreading the remaining sauce on the other side of fillets. Flip fillets one last time and cook 1 minute.
5. Remove and serve each fillet with a lemon wedge.

PER SERVING

Calories:227 | Fat: 9g | Sodium:405mg | Carbohydrates: 0g| Fiber: 0g| Sugar: 0g | Protein: 36g

Shrimp Ceviche

Prep time: 20 minutes, plus 4 hours to marinate| Cook time: 1 minute| Serves 12

- 3 pounds shrimp, peeled and deveined
- 1 cup (from about 8½) freshly squeezed lime juice
- 1 cup (from 8 medium) freshly squeezed lemon juice
- ⅓ cup (from 1 medium) freshly squeezed orange juice
- ¼ cup (from ½ medium) freshly squeezed grapefruit juice
- 2 large tomatoes, diced
- 1 large red onion, diced
- 1 bunch fresh cilantro, chopped
- 1 jalapeño pepper, diced
- 2 large cucumbers, peeled and diced
- 2 large avocados, peeled, seeded, and diced

1. Place a large pot of water over high heat. Bring to a boil.
2. Put the shrimp in the boiling water for 45 seconds. Quickly pour the contents of the pot over a strainer in the sink, and then immediately transfer the shrimp to ice-cold water; this stops the cooking. Drain when cooled.
3. Chop the shrimp into ½-inch pieces and put them in a large bowl.
4. Pour the lime juice, lemon juice, orange juice, and grapefruit juice over the shrimp, and toss to coat.
5. Add the tomatoes, red onion, cilantro, and jalapeño, and toss gently. Cover and marinate in the refrigerator for 4 hours.
6. Add the cucumbers and avocados before serving.

PER SERVING

Calories: 151 |carbs: 10.8g|fat: 3g|protein 21g

Spicy Grilled Shrimp Skewers

Prep time: 5 minutes | Cook time: 10 minutes| Serves 4

- 2 tablespoons minced scallions
- 1 teaspoon sriracha hot sauce
- 1 ½ tablespoons Thai sweet chili sauce
- 2 ½ tablespoons light mayonnaise
- 40 large raw shrimp, peeled and deveined
- 2 teaspoons ground black pepper

1. Preheat grill to medium.
2. In a small bowl, mix scallions, hot sauce, chili sauce, and mayonnaise, stirring well.
3. Thread 5 shrimp on each of 8 metal skewers and sprinkle with pepper.
4. Grill shrimp skewers 6–8 minutes per side. Remove from grill, coat with sauce, and serve warm.

PER SERVING

Calories: 153| Fat: 5g | Sodium:283mg | Carbohydrates: 4g| Fiber: 0g| Sugar: 3g | Protein: 23g

Parmesan-Crusted Salmon

Prep time: 5 minutes | Cook time: 15 minutes| Serves 1

- 1 (4-ounce) salmon fillet
- 1 teaspoon Dijon mustard
- 1 ½ teaspoons mayonnaise
- ⅛ teaspoon salt
- ⅛ teaspoon ground black pepper
- 1 ½ tablespoons grated Parmesan cheese

1. Preheat broiler. Line a small baking sheet with parchment paper.
2. Place fillet on prepared baking sheet.
3. In a small bowl, stir together mustard and mayonnaise. Brush mustard mixture on one side of fillet. Season with salt and pepper, then top with cheese.
4. Broil for 8–10 minutes until cheese is lightly browned and fillet flakes easily with a fork. Serve hot.

PER SERVING

Calories: 238| Fat: 13g | Sodium: 721mg| Carbohydrates:1g | Fiber:0 g| Sugar:0 g | Protein:30 g

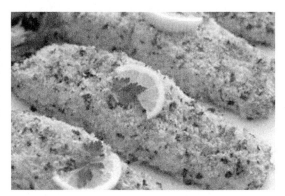

Tropical Shrimp Skewers

Prep time: 5 minutes | Cook time: 8 minutes| Serves 4

- 3 teaspoons minced garlic
- 2 tablespoons extra-virgin olive oil
- 2 tablespoons red wine vinegar
- 2 tablespoons chopped fresh parsley
- ½ teaspoon salt
- 2 pounds large shrimp, peeled and deveined
- 4 cups pineapple chunks
- 3 tablespoons shredded coconut

1. Preheat a gas or charcoal grill.
2. In a large bowl, combine garlic, oil, vinegar, parsley, and salt. Add shrimp and toss to coat.
3. Thread shrimp and pineapple alternately onto metal or wooden skewers. Transfer skewers to the grill and cook for 3–5 minutes per side until shrimp are pink.
4. Remove skewers from grill and sprinkle with coconut flakes before serving.

PER SERVING

Calories:297 | Fat: 10g | Sodium:282mg |
Carbohydrates: 25g| Fiber: 3g| Sugar: 18g | Protein: 28g

Honey-Garlic Shrimp

Prep time: 5 minutes, plus 15 minutes to marinate| Cook time: 2 minutes| Serves 4

- ¼ cup honey
- 2 tablespoons soy sauce (gluten-free, if desired) or liquid aminos
- 1 teaspoon garlic, minced
- ½ teaspoon ground ginger, minced
- 1 pound shrimp, peeled, deveined, and tails on
- 1 tablespoon coconut oil

1. In a large bowl, mix together the honey, soy sauce, garlic, and ginger. Transfer half of the mixture to another small bowl, and set aside.
2. Add the shrimp to the sauce in the large bowl, and toss to coat well. Marinate in the refrigerator for 15 minutes.
3. In a large skillet over medium-high heat, heat the coconut oil. Drain and discard any excess marinade from the shrimp, add the shrimp to the hot oil, and sear on both sides, about 1 minute per side, until the shrimp have slightly browned and the tails are pink. Remove from the heat.
4. Using a fork or tongs, rub the shrimp against the bottom of the skillet to collect the caramelized honey on the bottom of the pan.
5. Transfer to a plate, and drizzle with the remaining sauce. Divide among four plates and serve.

PER SERVING

Calories: 193 |carbs: 17.3g|fat: 4.5g|protein 20g

Garlic and Herb Shrimp

Prep time: 5 minutes, plus 2 hours to marinate| Cook time: 10 minutes| Makes 4 (4-ounce) servings

- 1 pound medium-size shrimp, peeled, deveined, and tails on
- 1 tablespoon extra-virgin olive oil
- 4½ teaspoons minced garlic
- 1 tablespoon granulated stevia
- 1 teaspoon ground paprika
- 1 teaspoon Italian seasoning
- 1 teaspoon dried basil

1. Put the shrimp, olive oil, lime juice, garlic, stevia, paprika, Italian seasoning, and basil in a large resealable bag. Massage the bag to ensure the shrimp are well coated. Marinate in the refrigerator for 2 hours.
2. Thread the shrimp onto skewers. If you are not using a rack, be sure to lightly spray the surface they are cooking on to prevent them from sticking.
3. To grill: Allow the barbecue to warm up to medium heat before placing the shrimp on the grill.
4. To broil: Set the oven rack about 8 inches from the broiler, line a broiler pan with aluminum foil, and arrange the shrimp skewers on it. Set your broiler to high and allow the oven to heat up a bit before placing the shrimp in it.
5. Cook the shrimp for 8 to 10 minutes, turning over once after 4 to 5 minutes. They are done when opaque with pink tails.
6. Serve warm.

PER SERVING

Calories: 130 |carbs: 4g|fat: 3.9g|protein 20g

Zoodle Shrimp Scampi

Prep time: 5 minutes | Cook time: 10 minutes| Serves 2

- 1 tablespoon olive oil
- 1 pound large shrimp, peeled and deveined
- 4 teaspoons minced garlic
- 1 teaspoon salt
- ½ teaspoon ground black pepper
- ¼ cup low-sodium chicken broth
- ¼ cup lemon juice
- 2 large zucchini, trimmed and spiralized
- 3 tablespoons grated Parmesan cheese
- ¼ cup chopped fresh Italian parsley

1. Heat oil in a large skillet over medium-low heat.
2. Add shrimp, garlic, salt, and pepper. Sauté for 4–6 minutes until shrimp start to turn pink.
3. Add broth, lemon juice, and zucchini noodles to the skillet. Increase heat to medium-high and bring to a boil. Cook for 1 minute or until shrimp are completely cooked and zucchini noodles are softened.
4. Sprinkle with cheese and parsley and serve immediately.

PER SERVING

Calories:349 | Fat: 15g | Sodium: 1,170mg|
Carbohydrates: 12g| Fiber: 4g| Sugar: 6g | Protein: 44g

Margarita Shrimp

Prep time: 5 minutes | Cook time: 45 minutes| Serves 4

- ½ tablespoon olive oil
- 1 pound large shrimp, peeled and deveined
- ¼ teaspoon ground cumin
- 4 cloves garlic, peeled and minced
- ¼ teaspoon crushed red pepper flakes
- ¼ teaspoon salt
- ¼ teaspoon ground black pepper
- 2 ounces tequila
- 2 tablespoons lime juice

1. Heat oil in a large skillet or wok over medium-high heat.
2. Season shrimp with cumin, garlic, red pepper flakes, salt, and black pepper, then add to hot oil and cook about 2 minutes per side.
3. Add tequila and cook another 30–40 seconds. Remove and drizzle with lime juice before serving.

PER SERVING

Calories: 114| Fat: 2g | Sodium:156mg |
Carbohydrates:0g | Fiber: 0g| Sugar: 0g | Protein: 24g

Chili Lime Salmon Pouches

Prep time 10 minutes | Cook time 15 minutes| Serves 4

- 1 medium wild salmon filet, approximately 1lb (450g)
- 2 large limes, sliced into ¼-inch (.5cm) slices (reserve ⅓ of each lime)
- 2 tsp chili powder
- ½ tsp salt
- 1 tsp ground cilantro

1. Preheat the oven to 400°F (204°C). Cut a piece of parchment paper large enough to create a pouch for the salmon. Place the parchment on a large baking sheet.
2. Arrange enough lime slices on the parchment paper to create a bed for the salmon filet. Place the filet, scales-side-down, on top of the lime slices.
3. Squeeze the reserved lime over the filet, discard. Season the filet with the chili powder, salt, and cilantro. Place the remaining lime slices on top of the filet.
4. Fold the parchment paper over the salmon and crimp the edges to form a pouch. Bake for 15 minutes. Serve hot.

PER SERVING

Calories:165 |fat:7.2g|carbs: 0g| protein: 25g

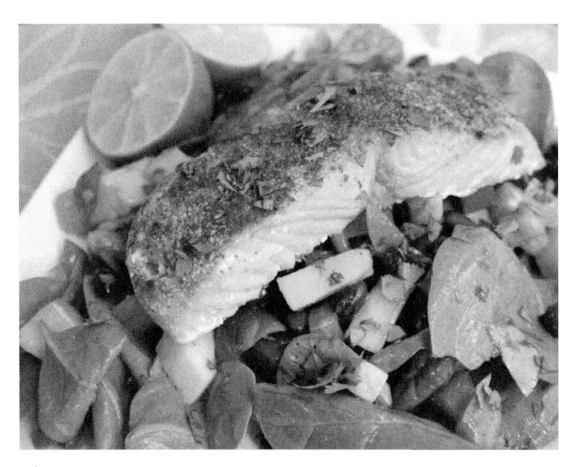

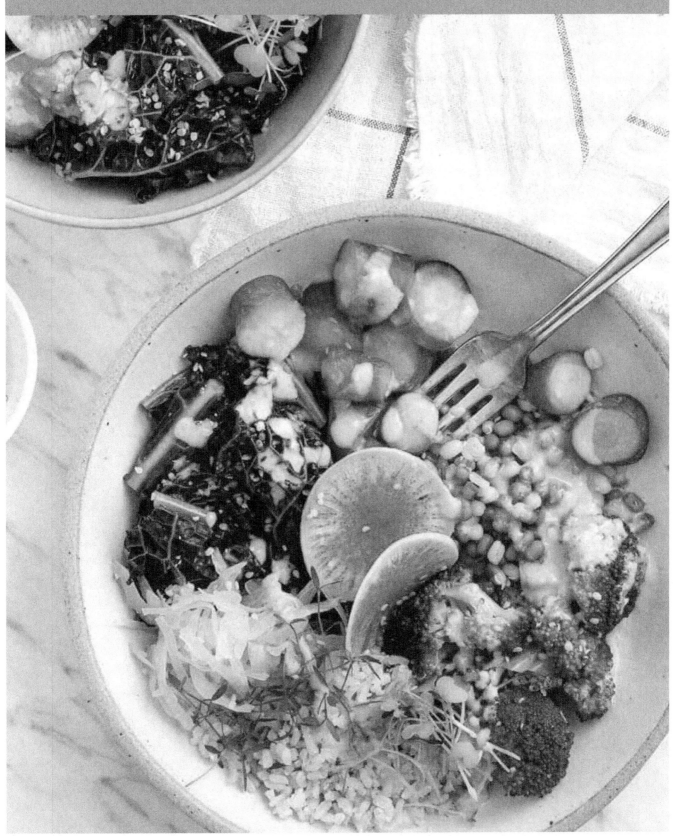

Chapter 8
Vegetarian and Vegan

Taco with White Bean Nachos

Prep time: 15 minutes | Cook time: 9 minutes | Serves 4

- 4 ounces (113g) unsalted corn tortilla chips
- ½ tablespoon olive oil
- 1 green bell pepper, seeded and diced
- 1 (15-ounce) can low-sodium white beans, drained and rinsed
- ½ tablespoon taco seasoning
- 1 teaspoon tomato paste
- 1 tablespoon water
- 2 tablespoons all-purpose flour
- ⅓ cup 1% milk
- ½ cup shredded low-fat cheddar cheese
- 2 scallions, green parts only, finely chopped

1. Arrange the tortilla chips on a large plate and set aside.
2. Heat the oil in a large nonstick skillet over medium heat. Add the bell pepper and sauté until tender, 5 to 7 minutes.
3. Add the beans, taco seasoning, tomato paste, and 1 tablespoon of water and cook, stirring occasionally, until heated through. Remove from the heat and set aside.
4. In a small bowl, whisk together the flour and milk.
5. Melt the cheese in a small saucepan over medium-low heat. Add the milk and flour mixture and cook, stirring constantly, until thickened, 1 to 2 minutes. Remove from the heat.
6. Spoon the bean mixture over the tortilla chips, top with the cheese mixture, and sprinkle with the scallions. Serve immediately.

PER SERVING

Calories: 349 | Fat: 12 g | Protein: 15 g | Sodium: 378 mg | Fiber: 7 g | Carbohydrates: 46 g | Sugar: 1 g

Tomato Parmesan-Chickpea Rotini

Prep time: 15 minutes | Cook time: 26 minutes | Serves 4

- 8 ounces (374g) whole-grain rotini
- 1 (15-ounce) can chickpeas, drained, rinsed, and dried
- 1½ tablespoons olive oil, divided
- 3 tablespoons bread crumbs
- 1½ tablespoons dried oregano, divided
- 2 teaspoons Italian seasoning, divided
- 1 large shallot, minced
- 4 garlic cloves, minced
- 1 cup canned crushed tomatoes
- ½ cup 1% milk
- 2 teaspoons balsamic vinegar
- ½ cup grated reduced-fat Parmesan cheese

1. Preheat the oven to 375°F (190°C). Line a baking sheet with parchment paper.
2. Cook the rotini according to the package instructions. Drain and set aside.
3. In a large bowl, mix the chickpeas, 1 tablespoon of olive oil, the bread crumbs, 1 tablespoon of the oregano, and 1 teaspoon of the Italian seasoning. Spread out the chickpeas on the prepared baking sheet. Avoid overcrowding. Bake for 20 minutes, or until lightly golden. Let cool on the baking sheet on a wire rack.
4. While the chickpeas are in the oven, heat the remaining ½ tablespoon of olive oil in a nonstick skillet over medium heat. Add the shallot and sauté until tender. Add the garlic and sauté until golden, about 1 minute.
5. Add the crushed tomatoes, milk, balsamic vinegar, the remaining ½ tablespoon oregano, and 1 teaspoon Italian seasoning and cook, stirring occasionally, for 1 to 2 minutes. Reduce the heat to low and cook, stirring occasionally, until the sauce slightly thickens, about 4 minutes. Remove from the heat and stir in the chickpeas.
6. Divide the rotini equally between 4 bowls. Top with the chickpea mixture, sprinkle with the Parmesan cheese, and serve immediately.

PER SERVING

Calories: 407 | Fat: 11 g | Protein: 17 g | Sodium: 438 mg | Fiber: 10 g | Carbohydrates: 66 g | Sugar: 1 g

Quinoa Tomato and Chickpea Bowl

Prep time: 15 minutes | Cook time: 15 minutes | Serves 4

- 1½ cups quinoa
- 1 (15-ounce) can chickpeas, drained and rinsed
- 1 teaspoon olive oil
- ¾ teaspoon garlic powder
- ¼ teaspoon chili flakes
- 3 cups fresh baby spinach
- 4 teaspoons all-purpose flour
- 1 cup 1% milk
- 2 tablespoons chopped sun-dried tomatoes
- ½ cup grated reduced-fat Parmesan cheese
- Sea salt to taste
- Freshly ground black pepper to taste

1. Cook the quinoa according to the package instructions. Drain and set aside.
2. Put the chickpeas into a large saucepan, add enough water to cover them, and cook over medium heat until heated through, 5 to 10 minutes. Drain the chickpeas and set aside.
3. Heat the olive oil in a large nonstick skillet over medium heat. Add the garlic powder and chili flakes and cook for 30 seconds. Add the spinach and cook, stirring frequently, until it wilts.
4. In a small bowl, whisk together the flour and milk. Reduce the heat to medium-low, add the flour and milk mixture, and cook, stirring, until combined.
5. Add the chickpeas and sun-dried tomatoes and cook, stirring, until thickened, 2 to 4 minutes. Remove from the heat. Add the quinoa and Parmesan and stir until combined. Add the salt and pepper to taste.
6. Divide the mixture equally between 4 bowls and enjoy.

PER SERVING

Calories: 414 | Fat: 11 g | Protein: 19 g | Sodium: 364 mg | Fiber: 9 g | Carbohydrates: 61 g | Sugar: 2 g

Pesto Chili

Prep time: 5 minutes | Cook time: 10 minutes | Serves 4

- 1 tablespoon olive oil
- 2 medium carrots, peeled and diced
- 1 small yellow onion, peeled and chopped
- 1 (15-ounce) can diced tomatoes
- 1 teaspoon salt
- 1 teaspoon freshly ground black pepper
- 2 cups water
- 1 (15-ounce) can chickpeas, drained and rinsed
- 1 (15-ounce) can cannellini beans, drained and rinsed
- 1 (15-ounce) can kidney beans, drained and rinsed
- ½ cup pesto

1. Add 1 tablespoon oil, carrots, and onion to a large saucepan over high heat and cook 3–5 minutes or until carrots are tender.
2. Stir in tomatoes, salt, pepper, and water and bring to a boil. Add chickpeas and other cans of beans, cooking until heated through (about 3 minutes).
3. Divide into 4 equal portions, top with pesto, and serve.

PER SERVING

Calories: 537 | Fat: 39g | Protein: 11g | Sodium: 1,209mg | Fiber: 12g | Carbohydrates: 37g | Sugar: 6g

Meatless Cheddar Squash Casserole

Prep time: 15 minutes | Cook time: 50 minutes | Serves 10

- 4 cups sliced summer squash
- ½ cup chopped onion
- ½ cup water
- 35 buttery round crackers, crushed
- 1 cup shredded Cheddar cheese
- 2 large eggs
- ¾ cup skim milk
- 1 teaspoon salt
- ½ teaspoon freshly ground black pepper
- ¼ cup unsalted butter, melted

1. Preheat oven to 400°F.
2. Place squash, onion, and water in a large skillet over medium-high heat and cover. Cook 5 minutes or until squash is tender, then drain and set aside.
3. In a medium bowl, combine crackers and cheese until well blended.
4. Stir half the cracker mixture into cooked squash and onions, mixing well.
5. In a separate medium bowl, whisk eggs and milk until well blended. Add to cracker and squash mixture, along with salt, pepper, and melted butter, mixing well.
6. Spread into a greased 9" × 13" glass baking dish, and top with remaining half of cracker and cheese mix.
7. Bake 25 minutes or until lightly browned, then serve.

PER SERVING

Calories: 184 | Fat: 13g | Protein: 7g | Sodium: 423mg | Fiber: 1g | Carbohydrates: 10g | Sugar: 3g

Oregano Tofu Slices with Sriracha Mayo

Prep time: 10 minutes | Cook time: 20 minutes | Serves 4

- 1 (14-ounce) package extra-firm tofu, drained and pressed for 20 minutes
- 1 large egg
- ⅔ cup bread crumbs
- 1 tablespoon dried oregano
- 1 teaspoon chili powder
- ¼ teaspoon freshly ground black pepper
- ¼ teaspoon sea salt
- ½ cup low-fat mayonnaise
- ½ tablespoon sriracha
- 6 cups mixed greens

1. Cut the tofu into 16 equal slices and place on a plate. Set aside.
2. Preheat the oven to 400°F (205°C). Line a baking sheet with parchment paper.
3. In a shallow bowl, beat the egg. In another large bowl, mix the bread crumbs, oregano, chili powder, pepper, and salt.
4. Dip 1 slice of tofu in the egg, dredge it in the bread crumb mixture, and place it on the prepared baking sheet. Repeat with the rest of the tofu slices.
5. Bake for 20 minutes, or until golden brown, flipping the slices over after 10 minutes.
6. In a small bowl, mix the mayonnaise and sriracha.
7. Divide the mixed greens equally between 4 bowls and pair with the tofu slices. Divide the sauce into 4 small bowls and serve on the side for dipping.

PER SERVING

Calories: 257 | Fat: 13 g | Protein: 15 g | Sodium: 327 mg | Fiber: 3 g | Carbohydrates: 22 g | Sugar: 2g

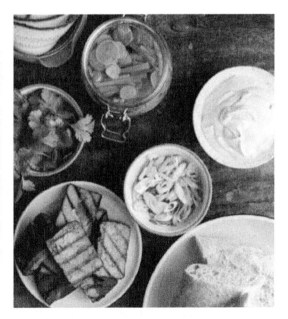

Brussels Sprouts in Pecan Butter

Prep time: 5 minutes | Cook time: 20 minutes| Serves 6

- Sea salt
- 1 pound (453g) Brussels sprouts
- 4 tablespoons (50g) butter
- 1 cup (125g) chopped pecans
- Freshly ground black pepper

1. Bring a large pot filled halfway with water to boil over high heat. Salt the water.
2. Meanwhile, trim the Brussels sprouts and mark an X in the bottom of each with a paring knife to promote even cooking.
3. Boil the Brussels sprouts in the salted water until tender, about 10 minutes.
4. Drain the water and cover the pot to keep the Brussels sprouts warm.
5. In a small sauté pan over medium heat, heat the butter until it turns nut brown, about 5 minutes. Add the pecans and toss until browned, 2 to 3 minutes.
6. Add the Brussels sprouts and toss to reheat, seasoning with salt and pepper to taste.
7. Divide the Brussels sprouts evenly among 6 airtight containers and seal.

PER SERVING

Calories: 232| Fat: 21g| Protein: 5g| Total Carbs: 10g| Net Carbs: 5g| Fiber: 5g| Sugar: 2g| Sodium: 72mg

Arugula Salad with Beets and Goat Cheese

Prep time: 5 minutes | Cook time: 5 minutes| Serves 3

- 3 tablespoons (45ml) extra-virgin olive oil
- 3 tablespoons (45ml) freshly squeezed lemon juice
- 3 tablespoons (45ml) Dijon mustard
- 1 tablespoon (15ml) pure maple syrup
- 3 beets (500g), peeled, chopped, and cooked
- 6 tablespoons (114g) crumbled feta cheese, divided
- 6 tablespoons (96g) walnut pieces, divided
- 9 cups (190g) arugula, divided

1. In a small bowl, mix together the olive oil, lemon juice, mustard, and maple syrup.
2. Into each of 3 airtight storage containers or jars, in this order, place a heaping 3 tablespoons of dressing topped by one-third of the chopped beets, 2 tablespoons of feta, 2 tablespoons of walnuts, and finally 3 cups of arugula. To serve, shake the jar or container before opening.

PER SERVING (1 MASON JAR)

Calories: 346| Fat: 27g| Protein: 10g| Total Carbs: 20g| Net Carbs: 15g| Fiber: 5g| Sugar: 15g| Sodium: 484mg

Baked Butternut Squash

Prep time: 5 minutes | Cook time: 50 minutes| Serves 4

- 1 pound (453g) butternut squash, chopped
- Sea salt
- Freshly ground black pepper
- ¼ teaspoon (0.6g) ground cinnamon
- ⅛ teaspoon (0.3g) chili powder
- 2 tablespoons (30ml) pure maple syrup
- 2 tablespoons (30ml) freshly squeezed lime juice
- 1 tablespoon (15ml) coconut oil

1. Preheat the oven to 350°F.
2. In a large bowl, mix the squash, salt, pepper, cinnamon, and chili powder.
3. Place the squash on a baking sheet or roasting pan, and drizzle with the maple syrup, lime juice, and coconut oil.
4. Bake, uncovered, for about 50 minutes, or until tender, stirring once halfway through baking. Remove from the oven and let cool.
5. Divide the squash evenly among 4 airtight storage containers and seal.

PER SERVING

Calories: 105| Fat: 4g| Protein: 1g| Total Carbs: 20g| Net Carbs: 16g| Fiber: 4g| Sugar: 8g| Sodium: 6mg

Thyme-Cauliflower Purée

Prep time: 5 minutes | Cook time: 10 minutes| Serves 6

- 3 cups (710ml) vegetable broth
- 2 medium (1.15kg) cauliflower heads, chopped into florets
- 3 garlic cloves (15g), minced
- 2 tablespoons (30ml) extra-virgin olive oil
- 2 tablespoons (30ml) coconut oil
- 1 tablespoon (2.4g) chopped fresh thyme
- 1 teaspoon (6g) sea salt, plus more for seasoning
- ¼ teaspoon (0.5g) freshly ground black pepper, plus more for seasoning

1. In a large stockpot, bring the broth to a boil and add the cauliflower.
2. Reduce the heat and simmer for 10 minutes.
3. Remove the cauliflower from the heat. Using a slotted spoon and reserving the broth, remove the cauliflower from the broth and transfer to a food processor.
4. Add the garlic, olive oil, coconut oil, thyme, salt, and pepper, and process until puréed. If you want the mixture even, smoother, add a few tablespoons of the hot broth and purée until smooth.
5. Season with additional salt and pepper. Let cool.
6. Divide the purée evenly among 6 airtight storage containers, and add a protein of your choice to make a complete meal.

PER SERVING (1 CONTAINER)

Calories: 150| Fat: 10g| Protein: 7g| Total Carbs: 12g| Net Carbs: 7g| Fiber: 5g| Sugar: 5g| Sodium: 752mg

Ginger-Garlic Tofu and Asparagus
Prep time: 15 minutes | Cook time: 29 minutes | Serves 4

- 1 (14-ounce) package extra-firm tofu, drained and pressed for 20 minutes
- 1½ tablespoons olive oil, divided
- 4 tablespoons corn starch, divided
- 12 asparagus spears, trimmed and cut into bite-size pieces
- 1 cup chopped mushrooms
- ½ cup low-sodium soy sauce
- 3 tablespoons honey
- 1 teaspoon minced fresh ginger
- 2 teaspoons minced garlic
- 4 scallions, green parts only, finely chopped

1. Cut the tofu into ½-inch pieces. In a large bowl, toss the tofu with ½ tablespoon of olive oil. Add 2 tablespoons of cornstarch and toss until evenly combined.
2. Heat ½ tablespoon of olive oil in a large nonstick skillet over medium-high heat. Add the tofu and cook, flipping the tofu every 2 to 3 minutes, until slightly browned, 8 to 10 minutes total. Transfer to a bowl and set aside.
3. In the same skillet, heat the remaining ½ tablespoon of oil over medium heat. Add the asparagus and cook for 5 to 6 minutes. Add the mushrooms and cook for 1 minute. Remove the pan from the heat.
4. While the asparagus is cooking, in a small saucepan, combine the soy sauce, honey, ginger, garlic, and ¾ cup water and bring to a boil over medium-high heat.
5. In a small bowl, mix the remaining 2 tablespoons of cornstarch and 1¼ cups of water. Add it to the sauce and mix well. Reduce the heat to low and cook until it reaches the desired thickness, 8 to 10 minutes. Remove from the heat.
6. Add the tofu to the asparagus, pour in the sauce, and stir well.
7. Divide the mixture equally between 4 bowls and garnish with the scallions. Serve immediately.

PER SERVING

Calories: 255 | Fat: 11 g | Protein: 15 g | Sodium: 1,161 mg | Fiber: 3g | Carbohydrates: 29 g | Sugar: 1 g

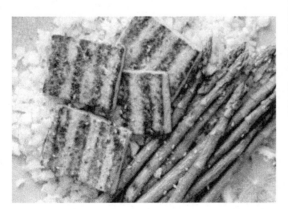

Stir-Fried Asparagus with Shiitake Mushrooms
Prep time: 5 minutes | Cook time: 10 minutes | Serves 3

- 8 ounces (225g) asparagus
- 6 ounces (170g) fresh shiitake mushrooms
- 1 tablespoon (15ml) sesame oil
- 2 teaspoons (8g) minced fresh garlic
- 1 teaspoon (4g) peeled and minced fresh ginger
- Crushed red chilies

1. Trim and discard the ends of the asparagus, and slice on the bias into 2-inch pieces. Wash and stem the mushrooms, and slice the caps into ½-inch slices.
2. In a large sauté pan or skillet over medium-high heat, heat the sesame oil.
3. Add the garlic and ginger, and stir-fry for a few seconds.
4. Add the mushrooms and asparagus, and stir-fry for 1 minute.
5. Add the crushed chilies and continue to stir-fry until the asparagus is nearly tender, about 3 minutes. Let cool.
6. Divide the vegetables evenly among 3 storage containers and seal.

PER SERVING

Calories: 106| Fat: 5g| Protein: 4g| Total Carbs: 15g| Net Carbs: 10g| Fiber: 5g| Sugar: 5g| Sodium: 140mg

Maple-Glazed Carrots
Prep time: 5 minutes | Cook time: 15 minutes | Serves 4

- Sea salt
- 2½ pounds (1.1kg) carrots
- 4 tablespoons (56g) butter
- Freshly ground black pepper
- ¼ cup (60ml) pure maple syrup
- 1 tablespoon (3.8g) chopped fresh parsley

1. Fill a large saucepan halfway with water and bring it to a boil over high heat. Salt the water.
2. Peel the carrots, and cut into 1-inch pieces.
3. Parboil the carrots in the salted water for about 2 minutes.
4. Drain the carrots. Wipe out the saucepan, melt the butter over medium heat, and sauté the carrots until nearly tender, 10 to 15 minutes.
5. Season with salt and pepper, and add the maple syrup. Garnish with the parsley.
6. Divide the carrots evenly among 4 airtight storage containers and seal.

PER SERVING

Calories: 266| Fat: 12g| Protein: 2g| Total Carbs: 40g| Net Carbs: 33g| Fiber: 7g| Sugar: 25g| Sodium: 273mg

Mushroom Halloumi Fajitas

Prep time: 10 minutes | Cook time: 20 minutes | Serves 4

- 1 green bell pepper, seeded and cut into slices
- 1 cup sliced grape tomatoes, divided
- ½ cup sliced mushrooms
- ⅓ small white onion, thinly sliced
- 7 ounces Halloumi, cut into strips
- ½ tablespoon olive oil
- 1 tablespoon fajita seasoning
- 8 (6-inch) corn tortillas
- 2 cups shredded lettuce

1. Preheat the oven to 450°F (235°C), line a large baking sheet with parchment paper, and set aside.
2. In a large bowl, add the bell pepper, ½ cup of tomatoes, mushrooms, onion, Halloumi, and olive oil and mix well. Sprinkle with the fajita seasoning, mix again, then arrange on the parchment paper, ensuring it is not overcrowded.
3. Bake in the oven for 12 to 15 minutes, or until golden brown. Remove the cooked Halloumi and continue to cook the vegetables for 5 minutes or until slightly tender.
4. To assemble, evenly divide the filling mixture into the tortillas and top with lettuce and the remaining ½ cup of tomatoes.

PER SERVING

Calories: 346 | Fat: 17 g | Protein: 18 g | Sodium: 200 mg | Fiber: 4 g | Carbohydrates: 18 g | Sugar: 1 g

Popeye'S Favorite Spinach

Prep time: 5 minutes | Cook time: 20 minutes | Serves 4

- 2 tablespoons (30ml) extra-virgin olive oil
- ½ large yellow onion (80g), finely chopped
- 2 (10-ounce) packages (600g) chopped frozen spinach, slightly thawed
- 2 garlic cloves (10g), crushed
- 3 large eggs
- Sea salt
- Freshly ground black pepper

1. In a medium saucepan over medium heat, heat the olive oil. Add the onion and sauté, stirring occasionally, for about 2 minutes.
2. Add the spinach and continue to cook uncovered for 2 more minutes, stirring regularly. Cover and continue cooking at a low temperature for about 15 more minutes, until the spinach is fully cooked.
3. Add the garlic and eggs, and stir just until the eggs are fully cooked. Season with salt and pepper. Remove from the heat and let cool.
4. Divide the spinach and eggs evenly among 4 airtight storage containers and seal.

PER SERVING (1 CONTAINER)

Calories: 154| Fat: 11g| Protein: 9g| Total Carbs: 8g| Net Carbs: 3g| Fiber: 5g| Sugar: 2g| Sodium: 154mg

Zucchini and Potato Bake

Prep time: 15 minutes | Cook time: 60 minutes| Serves 4

- 2 medium zucchini, sliced
- 4 medium potatoes, peeled and cut into large chunks
- 1 medium red bell pepper, seeded and chopped
- 1 clove garlic, minced
- ½ cup bread crumbs
- ¼ cup olive oil
- 1 teaspoon paprika
- 1 teaspoon salt
- 1 teaspoon freshly ground black pepper

1. Preheat oven to 400°F.
2. In a medium baking pan, toss all ingredients together, spreading evenly over the pan.
3. Bake 1 hour or until potatoes are tender, stirring occasionally.

PER SERVING

Calories: 349.65 | Fat: 14.9g | Protein: 7g | Sodium: 710mg | Fiber: 7.6g | Carbohydrates: 48g | Sugar: 7g

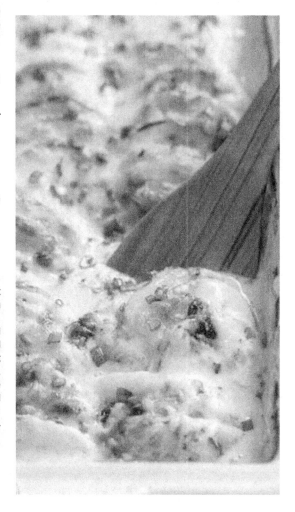

Vegetarian Buddha Bowl
Prep time: 5 minutes | Cook time: 30 minutes| Serves 4

- 2 large sweet potatoes (550g), peeled and cubed
- 1 large sweet onion (275g), sliced into large wedges
- 1 garlic clove (5g), minced
- Nonstick cooking spray
- Sea salt and black pepper
- 2 tablespoons (30ml) extra-virgin olive oil
- 2 tablespoons (30ml) freshly squeezed lemon juice
- 2 to 2½ teaspoons (10 to 12ml) honey
- 2 cups (312g) steamed broccoli florets, divided
- 1 (15.5-ounce) (425g) can chickpeas, rinsed and drained, divided
- 2 cups (140g) shredded kale, divided
- 1 medium avocado (150g), sliced, divided
- 1 cup (110g) shredded carrots, divided
- 2 tablespoons (20g) hemp hearts, divided

1. Preheat the oven to 400°F.
2. In a large bowl, combine the sweet potatoes, onion, and garlic. Spray well with cooking spray, and stir to combine, then season with salt and pepper. Spread out onto a baking sheet and bake for 25 to 30 minutes, or until the potatoes are tender.
3. Meanwhile, in a small bowl, whisk together the olive oil, lemon juice, and honey, and set aside.
4. Into each of 4 airtight storage containers, place half of the roasted sweet potatoes, then top each with ½ cup of steamed broccoli, ½ cup of chickpeas, ½ cup of kale, ¼ of the avocado, and ¼ cup of shredded carrots. Drizzle each Buddha bowl with 1 tablespoon of dressing, and season with salt and pepper. Sprinkle each bowl with ½ tablespoon of hemp hearts and seal.

PER SERVING

Calories: 414| Fat: 21g| Protein: 12g| Total Carbs: 47g| Net Carbs: 35g| Fiber: 12g| Sugar: 10g| Sodium: 74mg

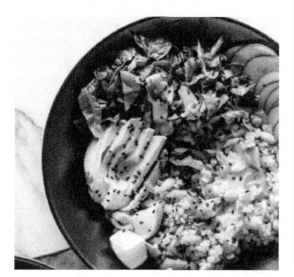

Veggie Fried Rice
Prep time: 5 minutes | Cook time: 30 minutes| Serves 6

- 2 cups (370g) basmati rice
- 1 teaspoon (1.2g) sea salt, plus more for seasoning
- 2 tablespoons plus 1 teaspoon (35ml) extra-virgin olive oil, divided
- 4 cups (950ml) water, plus 2 tablespoons (30ml), divided
- ½ medium onion (60g), finely chopped
- ½ red bell pepper (75g), finely chopped
- ½ yellow bell pepper (75g), finely chopped
- 1 celery stalk (38g), finely chopped
- 2 small tomatoes (120g), finely chopped
- Freshly ground black pepper

1. In a large stockpot, combine the rice, salt, 1 teaspoon of olive oil, and 4 cups of water. Bring to a boil.
2. Once boiling, turn down the heat to low, cover, and continue to simmer for 25 to 30 minutes, until the rice is tender and the water is absorbed.
3. Meanwhile, heat a large skillet over medium heat. Add the remaining 2 tablespoons of olive oil and the onion, and sauté for about 2 minutes.
4. Add the peppers, celery, and tomatoes and continue to sauté, stirring, for 2 more minutes. Season with salt and pepper.
5. Once the rice is ready, add in the vegetables and stir to combine. If needed, season with additional salt and pepper.
6. Divide the rice evenly among 6 airtight storage containers and seal.

PER SERVING (1 CONTAINER)

Calories: 270| Fat: 4g| Protein: 5g| Total Carbs: 53g| Net Carbs: 51g| Fiber: 2g| Sugar: 2g| Sodium: 324mg

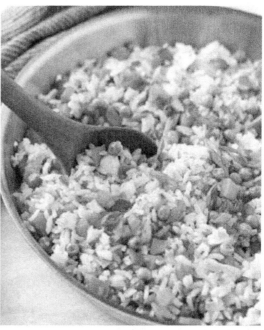

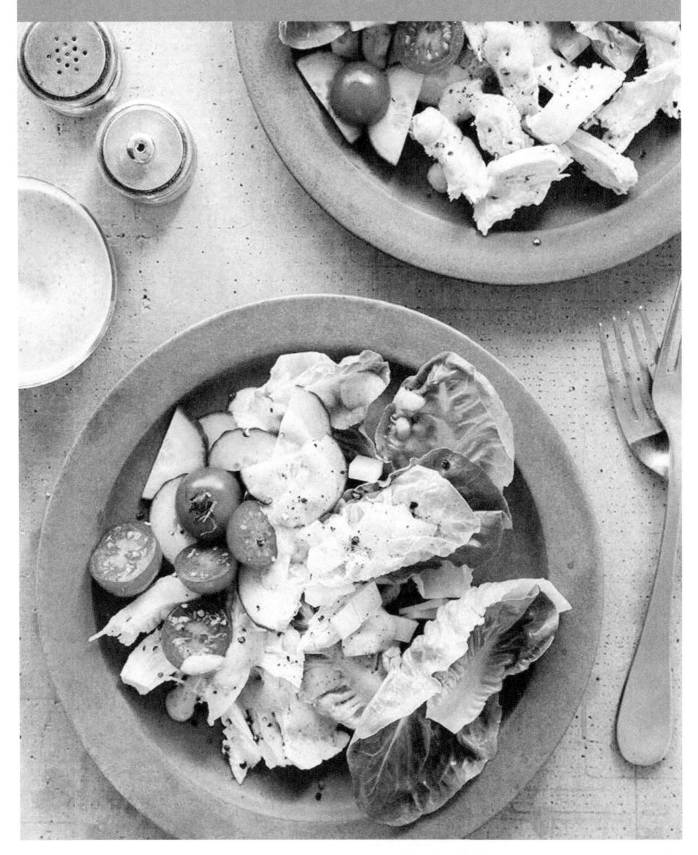

Chapter 9
Salads

Mediterranean Super Salad
Prep time: 5 minutes | Cook time: 5 minutes| Serves 1

- 1.5 cup quinoa
- 1 tsp olive oil
- ½ red onion, finely chopped
- 2 tbsp mint (fresh or dried) and roughly chopped
- 16oz of Puy or red lentils rinsed and drained – you can buy the dried lentils but you need to leave them to soak over night.
- ¼ cucumber (skin off and diced)
- 4oz crumbled feta cheese
- Zest and juice of 1 orange
- 1 tbsp red or white wine vinegar

1. Cook the quinoa in a large pan of boiling water for 10-15 minutes until soft, drain and set aside to cool.
2. Fry the onion in the oil over a medium heat.
3. Stir together with the quinoa, lentils, cucumber, feta, orange zest, chopped mint and juice and vinegar.
4. Best served chilled!
5. For the meat fans, cooked chicken or lamb would be a delicious addition to this dish!

PER SERVING

Calories: 290 | protein: 15g|carbs: 35g|fat: 10g

Hunked Up Halloumi
Prep time: 5 minutes | Cook time: 5 minutes| Serves 4

- 2 tbsp white wine vinegar
- 2 tsp olive oil
- ½ red onion thinly sliced
- Handful of rocket leaves
- ½ juiced lemon
- Handful of green/black olives
- 16oz of sliced halloumi cheese
- 1 tbsp mayonnaise
- ½ chopped cucumber
- A pinch of pepper

1. Preheat the grill.
2. Lightly drizzle a baking tray with 1 tsp olive oil before grilling for 5 minutes, turning until browned and crisp on the edges.
3. Add the chopped olives, rocket, cucumber and red onion into a bowl and mix with 1 tsp olive oil and lemon juice.
4. Season with pepper and stir in the mayonnaise (optional).
5. Serve alone or with crusty brown pitta breads for an Aegean twist!

PER SERVING

Calories: 461 | protein: 29g|carbs: 3g|fat: 37g

Roasted Beetroot, Goats' Cheese and Egg Salad
Prep time: 5 minutes | Cook time: 5 minutes| Serves 1

- 8oz cooked chopped beet root (not in vinegar)
- 2 tbsp olive oil
- Juice from 1 orange
- 2 eggs
- 1 tsp white wine vinegar
- 2 tbsp crème fraîche
- 1 tsp Dijon mustard
- A few stalks of dill, finely chopped (fresh or dried)
- Handful of walnuts
- 4oz crumbled goats cheese
- A pinch of salt and pepper

1. Preheat oven to (200°C/400°F/Gas Mark 6).
2. Place the beetroot onto the lightly oiled baking tray with the juice from the orange, sprinkle with salt and pepper.
3. Roast for 20-25 minutes, turning them once whilst they're baking. If they start to dry out, add a little more olive oil.
4. Meanwhile, put the eggs in boiling water. Turn down the heat and simmer for 8 minutes (4 minutes if you like your yolks runny) then run under cold water to cool. Peel and halve.
5. Mix the remaining oil, crème fraîche, mustard, a tsp of white wine vinegar and chopped dill together. This is the dressing for your lettuce.
6. Serve the salad with the beetroot and goats cheese crumbled over the top and walnuts sprinkled throughout

PER SERVING

Calories: 363 | protein: 11g|carbs: 18g|fat: 28g

Spicy Mexican Bean Stew
Prep time: 5 minutes | Cook time: 5 minutes| Serves 4

- 8oz canned chick peas, drained
- 8oz canned cannellini beans, drained
- 8oz of tinned chopped tomatoes
- 2 tbsp olive oil
- 1 chopped red onion
- 6oz of sliced chorizo
- 3 red chopped chillis
- 1 tbsp paprika

1. Heat a large pan on a medium heat with 1 tbsp olive oil, and cook the onion and chorizo for 5 minutes until lightly golden.
2. Tip in the chickpeas with the cannellini beans and stir until heated through.
3. Add the tin of chopped tomatoes and paprika and cover to let simmer for 5-10 minutes.
4. Serve - recommended with crusty brown bread, couscous or brown rice for a winter warmer!

PER SERVING

Calories: 395 | protein: 20g|carbs: 45g|fat: 15g

The Sailor Salad

Prep time: 5 minutes | Cook time: 5 minutes | Serves 4

- 1 bag of chopped spinach (fresh)
- 8oz of lean grilled chopped turkey breast (or turkey deli meat already cooked)
- 1 tbsp real bacon bits (you can cut up bacon and grill this yourself or buy the pre-packaged stuff)
- 2 diced hard-boiled eggs
- 4oz baby potatoes
- 1 deseeded and sliced red, yellow and green pepper
- 1 avocado peeled and sliced (do this near to the end or it will start to turn brown)
- 1 tbsp balsamic vinegar
- A pinch of salt and pepper

1. Boil a medium sized pan of water on a high heat and add the halved new potatoes, cooking for 15-20 minutes or according to packaging guidelines.
2. Combine the meats (once grilled and chopped if you're doing this yourself) with the spinach and peppers in a serving bowl.
3. Drain the potatoes and let cool whilst placing a small pan to boil for the eggs. Cook for 8 minutes for medium-boiled or 10 minutes for hard-boiled eggs.
4. Run the eggs under a cold tap and peel. Dice and add to your salad (here's where you can peel the avocado and add this).
5. Stir through with balsamic vinegar and salt and pepper to taste.

PER SERVING

Calories: 220 | protein: 20g|carbs: 13g|fat: 10g

Anabolic Avocado and Chicken Salad

Prep time: 5 minutes | Cook time: 5 minutes | Serves 1

- 1 chicken breast
- Handful of watercress
- Handful of baby spinach
- Handful of rocket
- ½ peeled and sliced avocado
- 1 chopped beef tomato
- ¼ sliced cucumber
- 2 tbsp of olive oil

1. Heat some olive oil on a medium heat in a griddle pan.
2. Grill the chicken breast for about 10 minutes each side or until cooked through.
3. Cut the chicken breasts into chunks and serve with the watercress, spinach, rocket, tomato and sliced avocado.
4. Finish off the salad by drizzling over olive oil.

PER SERVING

Calories: 389 | protein: 36g|carbs: 12g|fat: 14g

Muscle Building Steak and Cheese Salad

Prep time: 5 minutes | Cook time: 5 minutes | Serves 2

- 8oz frying beef steak
- 1 chopped red onion
- 1 teaspoon of crushed garlic
- Handful of baby spinach
- Handful of watercress
- Handful of lettuce
- 4 chopped baby tomatoes
- 2 tbsp of balsamic vinegar
- 1 tbsp olive oil
- 2oz of blue cheese
- A pinch of salt and pepper

1. Sprinkle salt and pepper over the steak.
2. Add a tbsp of olive oil to a griddle pan on a high heat.
3. Place the steak in the pan and cook 8 minutes in total, turning the steak half way through. Take the steak off the pan and allow to cool.
4. Cut the steak into 2cm strips, then place back into the pan and cook for a further minute on a medium heat.
5. Get a bowl and add the chopped tomatoes, watercress, baby spinach, lettuce, garlic and onions. Place the steak strips in the bowl along with the vinegar and a tbsp of olive oil. Mix everything together and grate the blue cheese over the top.

PER SERVING

Calories: 308 | protein: 34g|carbs: 15g|fat: 14g

Egg Salad

Prep time: 5 minutes | Cook time: 20 minutes | Serves 4

- 8 large eggs
- ½ cup low-fat mayonnaise
- 1 teaspoon mustard
- ¼ cup chopped green onion
- ¼ teaspoon salt
- ¼ teaspoon freshly ground black pepper
- ¼ teaspoon paprika

1. Place eggs in a medium saucepan and add cold water until eggs are covered by 1" water.
2. Bring water to a boil, then immediately remove pan from heat. Cover and let eggs cook 10-12 minutes, then immediately drain and cool under running cold water.
3. Peel eggs, chop, and mix with mayonnaise, mustard, onion, and seasonings.

PER SERVING

Calories: 176 | Fat: 12g | Protein: 13g | Sodium: 559mg | Fiber: 0g | Carbohydrates: 5g | Sugar: 3g

Strength Chicken and Sesame Salad

Prep time: 5 minutes | Cook time: 5 minutes| Serves 2

- 2 chicken breasts
- 3 tbsp of sesame oil
- 2 tsp of grated ginger
- 1 crushed garlic clove
- 1 chopped red chilli
- 1 diced red onion
- Handful of basil leaves
- Handful of coriander leaves
- 1 cup of baby spinach leaves
- 1 tsp of sesame seeds
- 4 chopped almonds
- 1 peeled and sliced mandarin

1. Pre-heat the grill.
2. Add 2 tbsp sesame oil, chopped red chilli, crushed garlic and ginger into a bowl. Mix all the ingredients together.
3. Make a few deep cuts into the chicken breast and leave them to marinate in the mixture for roughly 3 hours.
4. Add the spinach leaves, coriander leaves, basil leaves, red onion, chopped almonds and sesame seeds to a bowl and mix together.
5. Remove the chicken and rub over the last of the marinade and grill for 10 minutes each side or until fully cooked.
6. Cut the chicken into strips and add to the salad bowl.
7. Add the mandarin to the bowl and drizzle 1 tbsp of sesame oil over the salad and serve

PER SERVING

Calories: 430 | protein: 20g|carbs: 16g|fat: 15g

Sizzling Salmon Salad

Prep time: 5 minutes | Cook time: 5 minutes| Serves 1

- 6oz fillet salmon
- 6 cherry tomatoes
- 1 cup of couscous
- 3 stems of asparagus (chop off the very end of the base but leave the rest intact)
- 2oz of diced low-fat mozzarella cheese
- 1 bell pepper sliced
- 1 tbsp balsamic vinegar
- 1 tbsp olive oil
- A pinch of salt and pepper

1. Preheat the grill.
2. Layer the couscous with boiling water from the kettle (about 1cm over the top of the couscous, cover and leave to steam)
3. Grill salmon for 10-15 minutes or until cooked through. Place to one side.
4. Uncover the couscous and stir through with a fork to break up the grains.
5. Now just add your pepper, mozzarella and halved cherry tomatoes to the couscous.

6. You will need to grill your asparagus for 3-4 minutes, turning every so often until lightly browned around the surface.
7. Once the asparagus is ready, place it along with the salmon on the bed of couscous and drizzle with olive oil and balsamic vinegar.
8. Salt and pepper to taste.

PER SERVING

Calories: 521 | protein: 46g|carbs: 24g|fat: 27g

The Sweet Sailor Salad

Prep time: 5 minutes | Cook time: 5 minutes| Serves 4

- 1 cup raw spinach leaves
- 7oz lean grilled chopped turkey breast
- 1 tbsp grilled real bacon bits
- 2 eggs (free range)
- 4oz of chopped sweet potatoes
- 1 deseeded and sliced red, yellow and green pepper
- 1 avocado peeled and sliced (do this near to the end or it will start to turn brown)
- Sprinkle of salt and pepper

1. Bring a pan of water to the boil on a high heat and add the chopped potatoes.
2. Cook for 15-20 minutes or according to packaging guidelines.
3. Combine the cooked meats with the spinach and peppers.
4. Drain the potatoes and leave to cool whilst placing a small pan of water to boil for the eggs.
5. Add the eggs once boiling and cook for 8 minutes for a medium-boiled and 10 minutes for a hard-boiled egg.
6. Run the eggs under a cold tap and peel.
7. Chop in half and add to your salad (here's where you can peel the avocado and add this).
8. Stir through your choice of olive oil, red/white wine vinegar and salt and pepper to taste.

PER SERVING

Calories: 220 | protein: 20g|carbs: 13g|fat: 10g

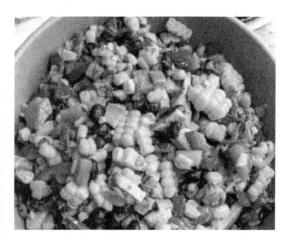

Muscle Building Steak and Balsamic Spinach Salad

Prep time: 5 minutes | Cook time: 5 minutes| Serves 2

- 8oz frying beef steak
- 1 chopped red onion
- 1 tsp of crushed garlic
- 1/4 cup baby spinach
- 1/4 cup watercress
- 4 cherry tomatoes, halved
- 2 tbsp of balsamic vinegar
- 2 tbsp olive oil
- Sprinkle of salt and pepper

1. Sprinkle salt and pepper over steak.
2. Add a tbsp of olive oil to a griddle pan and heat on a high temperature.
3. Place the steak in the pan and cook for 8 minutes in total, turning the steak half way through.
4. Remove the steak from the pan and rest for 3 minutes.
5. Cut it into 2cm strips.
6. Get a bowl and add the chopped tomatoes, watercress, baby spinach, garlic and onions.
7. Place the steak strips in the bowl along with the vinegar and a tbsp of olive oil. Mix together.
8. Plate up and serve.

PER SERVING

Calories: 308 | protein: 34g|carbs: 15g|fat: 14g

Spicy Black Beans and Quinoa

Prep time 10 minutes | Cook time 25 minutes| Serves 8

- 1 jalapeño pepper, seeds and stem removed, finely diced
- 2 tsp minced garlic
- 2 cups low fat chicken broth
- 1½ cups uncooked white quinoa, rinsed 3 to 4 times
- 1 15oz (420g) can diced fire-roasted tomatoes, not drained
- ½ tsp chipotle powder
- 1 tsp ground cumin
- 1 tsp onion powder
- 1 tsp paprika
- 1 15oz (420g) can black beans, drained and rinsed
- 1 cup frozen corn kernels

1. Spray a large skillet with non-stick cooking spray and place over medium heat. Add the jalapeño and garlic to the pan and cook for 1 minute, or until the garlic starts to soften and becomes fragrant. Stir frequently.
2. Add the chicken broth, quinoa, tomatoes, chipotle powder, cumin, onion powder, and paprika to the pan. Increase the heat to high and bring to a boil, stirring constantly. As soon as the mixture reaches a boil, reduce the heat to low, cover, and cook for 15 minutes.
3. Add the black beans and corn. Stir, cover, and continue to cook for an additional 4 to 5 minutes, or until the quinoa is tender. Serve hot.

PER SERVING

Calories:154 |fat:2.4g|carbs: 28.5g| protein: 5.6g

Protein Packed Egg and Bean Salad

Prep time: 5 minutes | Cook time: 5 minutes| Serves 6

- 16oz of cooked black beans, drained and rinsed
- 16oz of cooked cannellini beans, drained and rinsed
- 16oz of cooked kidney beans, drained and rinsed
- 6 hard-boiled eggs, sliced
- 1 celery stick chopped
- ½ onion, chopped
- Handful of olives, sliced
- 3 tsp of hot pepper sauce
- ½ tsp of salt
- ¼ tsp of pepper
- 3 tsp of Italian salad dressing

1. Drain the beans, then rinse, and finally drain again.
2. Combine celery, olives, onions, salad dressing, seasonings, and beans. Carefully mix. Refrigerate for at least 2 hours, preferably overnight.
3. When ready to serve. Drain off the salad dressing first, then add eggs.
4. Carefully mix so as not to mash the beans.
5. Serve.

PER SERVING

Calories: 366 | protein: 15g|carbs: 30g|fat: 14g

Avocado Southwestern Salad

Prep time: 5 minutes | Cook time: 10 minutes| Serves 4

- ¼ cup olive oil
- ¼ cup lime juice
- ½ teaspoon ground cumin
- 1 teaspoon salt
- 1 teaspoon freshly ground black pepper
- 2 bags (about 12 cups) romaine lettuce
- 2 medium avocados, peeled, pitted, and cubed
- 1 (15.5-ounce) can pinto beans, drained and rinsed
- 1 cup cooked corn kernels
- ½ medium red onion, peeled and diced
- ½ cup chopped fresh cilantro

1. For dressing: Whisk together oil, lime juice, cumin, salt, and pepper until emulsified.
2. For salad: Toss lettuce, avocados, beans, corn, onion, and cilantro in a large bowl.
3. Mix dressing with salad and serve.

PER SERVING

Calories: 274 | Fat: 15g | Protein: 8g | Sodium: 882mg | Fiber: 9g | Carbohydrates: 32g | Sugar: 5g

Chickpea Salad

Prep time: 5 minutes | Cook time: 10 minutes| Serves 4

- 1 (19-ounce) can chickpeas, drained and rinsed
- 1 stalk celery, chopped
- ½ medium onion, peeled and chopped
- 1 tablespoon mayonnaise
- 1 tablespoon lemon juice
- 1 teaspoon dried dill

1. In a medium bowl mash chickpeas with a fork.
2. Add all other ingredients, mix well, and refrigerate until ready to eat.

PER SERVING

Calories: 125 | Fat: 4.2g | Protein: 5.2g | Sodium: 33mg | Fiber: 4.7g | Carbohydrates: 17.4g | Sugar: 3.5g

Hasselback Sweet Potatoes with Spicy Crema

Prep time 10 minutes | Cook time 65 minutes| Serves 5

- 2lbs (1kg) sweet potatoes (look for round shapes, rather than oblong)
- Coconut oil cooking spray
- ½ tsp salt
- ⅓ cup nonfat Greek yogurt
- 3 tbsp jarred red enchilada sauce
- ½ tsp fresh-squeezed lime juice
- ¼ tsp powdered stevia

1. Preheat the oven to 400°F (204°C). Spray a medium baking dish with coconut oil cooking spray.
2. Slice the sweet potatoes crosswise, about three fourths of the way through. The slices should be approximately ¼-inch (.5cm) thick. Place the sliced sweet potatoes in the baking dish and lightly spray with the coconut oil cooking spray, and season with the salt.
3. Tightly cover the dish with aluminum foil and bake for 45 minutes. Uncover and bake for an additional 15 minutes. Remove from the oven and allow to cool for 10 minutes.
4. While the sweet potatoes cool, prepare the crema by combining the Greek yogurt, enchilada sauce, lime juice, and stevia in a medium bowl. Mix well to combine.
5. Drizzle the crema over top of the potatoes. Serve warm.

PER SERVING

Calories:151 |fat:0.4g|carbs: 34g| protein: 3.3g

Herby Tuna Steak

Prep time: 5 minutes | Cook time: 5 minutes| Serves 2

- 2x 8oz dolphin-friendly yellow fin tuna steaks
- 1 tbsp olive oil
- 2 lemon wedges
- 2 handfuls of flat-leaf parsley and 2 handfuls of coriander very roughly chopped
- 2 cloves of finely chopped garlic
- Handful chopped green olives
- 6 tbsp olive oil
- 2oz pine nuts or walnuts
- Juice of half a lemon

1. Your first job is the herby salad – mix the herbs with half of the chopped garlic, lemon juice and olive oil.
2. Crush the nuts in a tea towel or blend them up in your blender. Stir them in to the herbs.
3. Brush the tuna steaks with olive oil and sprinkle with salt and pepper.
4. Seal the tuna in the pan for one minute on each side (if you have a griddle pan or grill then you should place these against the lines to get that nice straight off the BBQ look and taste)
5. If you like your tuna less-pink cook for 2 minutes on each side for medium, 3 for medium well and 4 for well done (approximate times).
6. Once cooked serve straight away with your herby salad (pour this over as a dressing or on the side as an accompaniment)

PER SERVING

Calories: 578 | protein: 35g|carbs: 3g|fat: 48g

Healthy Quinoa Salad

Prep time: 5 minutes | Cook time: 20 minutes| Serves 4

- 1 cup (240ml) vegetable broth
- ½ cup (85g) quinoa, rinsed
- ½ red bell pepper (75g), chopped
- ½ medium onion (60g), chopped
- ¼ English cucumber (50g), peeled, seeded, and chopped
- 2 tablespoons (22g) finely chopped fresh mint
- Juice of ½ lime (30ml)
- Sea salt
- Freshly ground black pepper

1. In a medium saucepan, bring the vegetable broth to a boil.
2. Add the quinoa, cover, and reduce the heat to medium-low. Cook for about 15 minutes, or until all liquid is absorbed.
3. In a medium bowl, combine the quinoa, bell pepper, onion, cucumber, mint, lime juice, and olive oil. Season with salt and pepper, and mix well.
4. Divide the salad evenly among 4 airtight storage containers and seal.

PER SERVING

Calories: 165| Fat: 9g| Protein: 5g| Total Carbs: 18g| Net Carbs: 16g| Fiber: 2g| Sugar: 2g| Sodium: 194mg

Tuna and Super Spinach Salad

Prep time: 5 minutes | Cook time: 5 minutes| Serves 2

- 2x 4oz cans of tinned tuna in olive oil
- Handful of baby spinach
- 1 chopped red onion
- 2 chopped red or green peppers
- 1 tbsp olive oil
- 1 chopped red chilli
- 10 halved cherry tomatoes
- Handful of chopped black olives
- ½ iceberg lettuce chopped into slices

1. Get a bowl and mix all of the ingredients apart from the lettuce together before tossing and drizzling with olive oil.
2. Layer the salad onto your plate before topping with the tuna mixture.
3. Serve and enjoy.

PER SERVING

Calories: 302 | protein: 18g|carbs: 28g|fat: 13g

Greek Grilled Chicken Salad

Prep time: 5 minutes | Cook time: 20 minutes| Serves 4

- 2 (10-ounce) (566g) boneless, skinless chicken breasts
- Sea salt and black pepper
- 2 tablespoons (30ml) extra-virgin olive oil
- 2½ teaspoons (12.5ml) freshly squeezed lemon juice
- 2½ teaspoons (12.5ml) red wine vinegar
- 1½ tablespoons (7.5g) chopped fresh oregano
- 1 English cucumber (200g), chopped
- 8 ounces (250g) kalamata olives
- 2 tomatoes (200g), cut into slices
- ½ cup (30g) chopped fresh parsley
- ½ cup (80g) red onion
- 1 cup (113g) crumbled feta cheese, divided
- ½ head (313g) romaine lettuce, chopped, divided

1. Heat a grill to medium-high or preheat the broiler to high.
2. Season the chicken breasts with salt and pepper. Grill for 7 to 10 minutes on each side, or broil in a broiler pan 6 inches from the heat for 10 minutes on each side. Let cool completely, and cut into strips.
3. In a small bowl, whisk together the olive oil, lemon juice, vinegar, and oregano.
4. In a medium bowl, toss to combine the cucumber, peppers, olives, tomatoes, parsley, and onion, and season with pepper.
5. Into each of 4 mason jars, place about 2 teaspoons of dressing, one-quarter of the veggie mixture, ¼ cup of crumbled feta, and one-quarter of the lettuce and seal. To serve, shake to distribute the dressing and eat directly from the jar, or invert the jar's contents into a bowl.

PER SERVING

Calories: 443| Fat: 22g| Protein: 46g| Total Carbs: 18g| Net Carbs: 12g| Fiber: 6g| Sugar: 7g| Sodium: 123mg

Roasted Sweet Potato Medallions

Prep time 10 minutes | Cook time 55 minutes| Serves 4

- 2 large white or purple sweet potatoes, washed and peeled
- Coconut oil cooking spray
- 1 tsp salt
- Pinch of cinnamon
- ½ tsp ground chipotle powder
- ½ tsp paprika

1. Preheat the oven to 400°F (204°C). Generously spray a 9 x 13in (23 x 33cm) baking pan with coconut oil cooking spray.
2. Slice the potatoes crosswise into ½-inch (1.25cm) medallions. Place the medallions in a large bowl and lightly spray with coconut oil cooking spray.
3. Season the potatoes with the salt, cinnamon, chipotle powder, and paprika. Toss to evenly distribute the spices over the potatoes. Arrange the medallions in a single layer in the baking pan.
4. Roast for 40 to 50 minutes, flipping the potatoes halfway through the cooking time. The potatoes are done when they begin to brown and become soft in the center. Serve hot.

PER SERVING

Calories:150 |fat:0g|carbs: 33g| protein: 5g

Bulgur Wheat, Feta Cheese and Quinoa Salad

Prep time: 5 minutes | Cook time: 5 minutes| Serves 4

- 1/2 cup of bulgur wheat, uncooked
- 1/2 cup of cooked quinoa
- 16oz of chickpeas, drained
- 2oz of feta cheese, crumbled
- 1 cup cherry tomatoes, chopped
- ½ jar of pesto
- 3 tbsp of fresh lemon juice
- 2 tbsp of fresh parsley, minced
- 1/4 tsp of black pepper
- 1 onion, sliced thinly
- 2 cups of water, boiling

1. Mix bulgur wheat with boiling water in a large-sized bowl. Cover and set aside for half an hour before draining.
2. Add lemon juice and pesto. Stir using a whisk.
3. Combine pesto mixture, bulgur, quinoa, feta, tomatoes, green onions, chickpeas, pepper, parsley in a large bowl. Gently toss to mix well.
4. Serve

PER SERVING

Calories: 350 | protein: 15g|carbs: 50g|fat: 15g

Coconut Cayenne Smashed Sweet Potatoes

Prep time 30 minutes | Cook time 65 minutes| Serves 6

- 2lbs (1kg) sweet potatoes, washed and ends trimmed
- $\frac{1}{2}$ cup light coconut milk
- 2 tsp ground cinnamon
- $\frac{1}{2}$ tsp ground cayenne pepper

1. Preheat the oven to 400°F (204°C). Pierce the sweet potatoes with a fork and individually wrap in aluminum foil. Place directly on the oven rack and bake for 1 hour, turning the potatoes halfway through the baking time.
2. Remove the potatoes from the oven and allow to cool for 20 minutes. Once cooled, remove the foil and peel the skin from the potatoes.
3. In a large bowl, combine the peeled sweet potatoes, coconut milk, cinnamon, and cayenne pepper.
4. Using a fork or immersion blender, thoroughly smash the ingredients together until a smooth consistency is achieved, and no lumps remain. Serve warm.

PER SERVING

Calories: 139|fat:0.7g|carbs: 31.7g| protein: 2.1g

Carb Cutter Twice-Baked Potatoes

Prep time 10 minutes | Cook time 95 minutes| Serves 4

- 2 medium russet potatoes
- 1 cup broccoli florets, chopped
- 2 cups cauliflower florets
- $\frac{1}{2}$ cup unflavored coconut milk
- $\frac{1}{2}$ tbsp white vinegar
- 1 tbsp dried chives
- 1 tsp salt
- $\frac{1}{2}$ tsp ground black pepper
- 8 tbsp low fat shredded cheddar cheese

1. Preheat the oven to 400°F (204°C). Pierce the potatoes with a fork, individually wrap in aluminum foil, and place on the middle oven rack. Bake for 1 hour.
2. While the potatoes bake, fill a large pot with 1 inch (2.5cm) water, and place a steamer tray in the bottom of the pot. Place the broccoli and cauliflower in the pot, cover, and steam for 10 minutes. Use a slotted spoon to remove only the broccoli to a small bowl. Steam the cauliflower for an additional 10 minutes.
3. Remove the potatoes from the oven and allow to cool for 15 minutes. Once cooled, unwrap the potatoes and remove the foil, slice lengthwise, and use a small spoon to scoop the flesh out into a large bowl. Reserve the skins and set the bowl aside.
4. Add the cooked cauliflower to the potato, and use a fork or immersion blender to thoroughly mash the ingredients together. Add the coconut

milk, vinegar, chives, salt, and black pepper, and continue to mash until all ingredients are well incorporated and smooth texture is achieved.
5. Scoop the cauliflower and potato mixture into the reserved skins. Top each with the broccoli and 2 tbsp cheddar cheese. Place back in the oven and bake for an additional 15 minutes. Serve hot.

PER SERVING

Calories:118 |fat:1.2g|carbs: 24.5g| protein: 4.4g

Baked Zucchini Fries

Prep time 10 minutes | Cook time 25 minutes| Serves 2

- 2 large zucchini, ends trimmed and sliced lengthwise into 8 wedges
- $\frac{1}{4}$ cup liquid egg whites
- $\frac{1}{2}$ cup grated parmesan cheese
- $\frac{1}{2}$ tsp garlic powder
- $\frac{1}{2}$ tsp ground black pepper

1. Preheat the oven to 425°F (218°C). Line a 9 x 13-inch (23 x 33cm) baking sheet with aluminum foil. Place an oven-safe cooling rack on top of the foil, and spray with non-stick cooking spray.
2. Pour the egg whites into a small bowl. In a separate small bowl, combine the parmesan cheese, garlic powder, and black pepper. Mix well to combine.
3. Dip the zucchini wedges in the egg whites, then dredge them in the parmesan mixture. Place the fries on the cooling rack.
4. Bake for 18 to 20 minutes, or until the fries turn golden brown. Serve hot.

PER SERVING

Calories:74 |fat:3.3g|carbs: 5.1g| protein: 77g

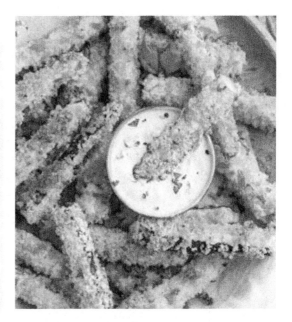

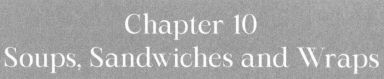

Chapter 10
Soups, Sandwiches and Wraps

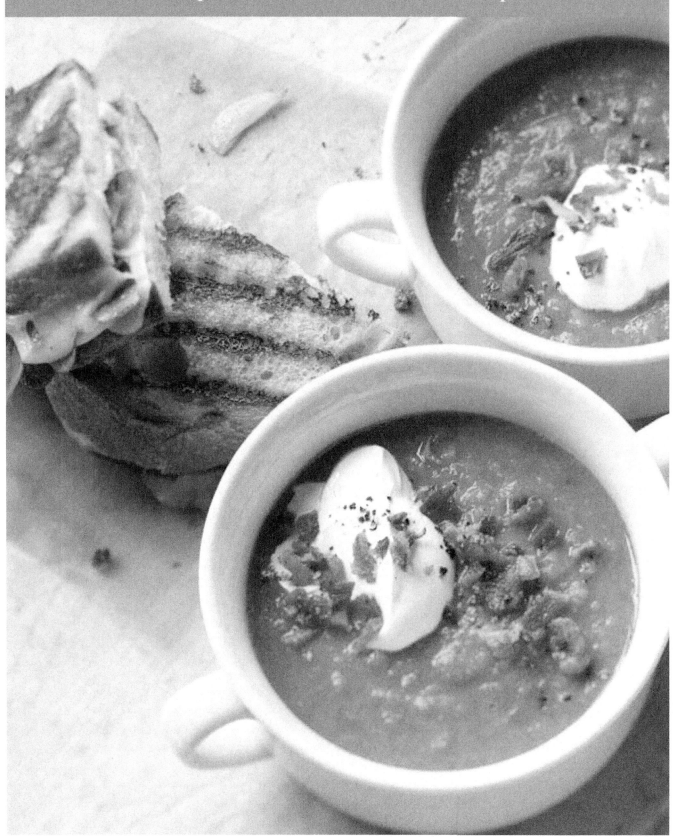

Guacamole Chicken Lettuce Wraps

Prep time: 5 minutes | Cook time: 7 minutes | Serves 4

- 1 pound ground chicken
- 1 cup Cowboy Caviar or salsa with black beans and corn
- 8 large soft leaves Boston lettuce
- 3 tablespoons guacamole

1. Spray a medium skillet with nonstick cooking spray and heat over medium-high heat. Add ground chicken to the skillet. Sauté, using a wooden spoon to break up meat, until no pink remains, about 5 minutes.
2. Stir in Cowboy Caviar or salsa, reduce heat to medium-low, and cook for another 2 minutes.
3. Lay lettuce leaves on a flat surface. Fill each leaf with about ¼ cup chicken mixture and top with guacamole. Roll filled lettuce into cylinders and serve immediately.

PER SERVING

Calories: 308 | Fat: 10.5 g | Protein: 22 g | Sodium: 131 mg | Fiber: 2 g | Carbohydrates: 35 g | Sugar: 30 g

Cheese and Creamy Potato Soup

Prep time: 10 minutes | Cook time: 65 minutes | Serves 4

- 2 medium russet potatoes
- 1 small head cauliflower, cored, outer leaves removed, and chopped
- 1½ cups low-sodium chicken broth
- 1½ cups whole milk
- ½ cup sour cream
- ½ cup shredded Cheddar cheese
- 6 tablespoons chopped chives
- 1 teaspoon salt
- 1 teaspoon ground black pepper
- 3 slices bacon, cooked and crumbled

1. Preheat oven to 400°F (205°C).
2. Place potatoes on a baking sheet and bake 1 hour. Cool 10 minutes, then cut potatoes in half. Scoop the flesh from each half and roughly dice. Set aside.
3. Place cauliflower in a steamer basket. In a medium saucepan, bring 1" of water to a boil. Place steamer basket in saucepan, cover, and reduce heat to medium-low. Steam cauliflower for 5 minutes.
4. Combine potatoes, broth, and milk in a large saucepan and bring to a boil over medium-high heat. Stir in cauliflower.
5. Remove from heat, then transfer soup to a blender and process until smooth (or use a handheld blender).
6. Return soup to pot and place over low heat and stir in sour cream, cheese, chives, salt, and pepper. Simmer 10 minutes, stirring frequently.
7. Top with bacon before serving.

PER SERVING

Calories: 186 | Fat: 9 g | Protein: 7 g | Sodium: 609mg | Fiber: 3 g | Carbohydrates: 19 g | Sugar: 3 g

Onion Cheddar Cauliflower Soup

Prep time: 10 minutes | Cook time: 25 minutes | Serves 2

- 2 tablespoons olive oil
- 1 small yellow onion, peeled and chopped
- 2 cloves garlic, minced
- 1 medium cauliflower head, rinsed and chopped
- 4 cups low-sodium chicken broth
- ½ cup grated Parmesan cheese

1. Heat oil in a large saucepan over medium heat and add onion and garlic.
2. After 5 minutes, add cauliflower and chicken stock, bringing to a boil.
3. Reduce heat and simmer 20 minutes or until cauliflower is soft.
4. Transfer mixture to a blender and blend in batches until smooth.
5. Return to pan, stir in Parmesan, and heat through before serving.

PER SERVING

Calories: 341 | Fat: 21 g | Protein: 17 g | Sodium: 670mg | Fiber: 6 g | Carbohydrates: 24g | Sugar: 7 g

Tomato and Basil Focaccia Sandwich

Prep time: 10 minutes | Cook time: 0 minute | Serves 2

- 2 tablespoons low-fat mayonnaise
- 2 tablespoons chopped fresh basil
- 2 tablespoons sun-dried tomatoes
- ¼ teaspoon crushed red pepper
- 8 ounces (227 g) sliced turkey
- 1 cup spinach leaves
- 4 slices focaccia bread

1. In a small bowl, mix mayonnaise, basil, tomatoes, and crushed red pepper. Divide the mixture in half.
2. Build sandwiches by layering the spread, turkey, and spinach leaves on two slices focaccia, and then topping with two slices.

PER SERVING

Calories: 421 | Fat: 13 g | Protein: 25 g | Sodium: 1,679 | Fiber: 1 g | Carbohydrates: 52g | Sugar: 3g

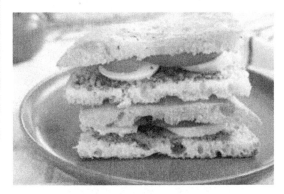

Taco Corn Chowder

Prep time: 5 minutes | Cook time: 35 minutes| Serves 4

- 2 tablespoons olive oil
- 8 cups frozen corn kernels, thawed
- 1 medium yellow onion, peeled and diced
- 1 tablespoon taco seasoning
- 1 teaspoon salt
- 6 cups low-sodium chicken broth
- ½ cup shredded pepper jack cheese

1. In a large pot over medium-high heat, heat oil. Add corn, onion, taco seasoning, and salt.
2. Sauté for 7–8 minutes until onion is soft.
3. Remove one-third of the mixture and set aside.
4. Add broth to the pot and bring to a boil. Reduce heat to medium-low and simmer for 15 minutes.
5. Remove from heat, then transfer soup to a blender and process until smooth (or use a handheld blender).
6. Return soup to pot and stir in the reserved corn mixture. Simmer over medium-low heat for 3 minutes.
7. Ladle soup into four bowls and top with cheese. Serve immediately.

PER SERVING

Calories: 412| Fat: 12g | Sodium:857mg | Carbohydrates: 67g| Fiber: 4g| Sugar: 12g | Protein: 13g

Wheat Pulled-Chicken BBQ Sandwiches

Prep time: 5 minutes | Cook time: 0 minute | Serves 1

- 4 ounces (113g) shredded slow-cooked chicken
- 2 tablespoons barbecue sauce (or any other sauce of your choice)
- 1 whole-wheat hamburger bun

1. In a medium bowl, mix chicken and sauce until chicken is coated completely. (It's best if chicken is heated.)
2. Place chicken on sandwich bun and serve.

PER SERVING

Calories: 316 | Fat: 3 g | Protein: 29 g | Sodium: 1,003 | Fiber: 4 g | Carbohydrates: 43g | Sugar: 14g

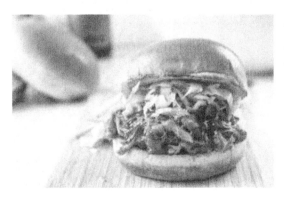

Black Bean Soup

Prep time: 15 minutes | Cook time: 4 hours 30 minutes| Serves 6

- 2 tablespoons olive oil
- 2 medium carrots, peeled and chopped
- 2 stalks celery, chopped
- 1 medium onion, peeled and chopped
- ¼ cup tomato paste
- 3 cloves garlic, minced
- 1½ teaspoons ground cumin
- 3 (15-ounce) cans black beans, drained and rinsed
- 1 cup frozen or canned corn
- 3 cups vegetable broth

1. Heat oil in a medium skillet over medium-high heat.
2. Add carrots, celery, and onion to the pan and cook 5 minutes, stirring occasionally.
3. Stir in tomato paste, garlic, and cumin and continue to cook 2 minutes, stirring frequently.
4. In a large slow cooker (at least 4 quarts), combine skillet mixture with beans, corn, and broth. Cook on high 4 hours.
5. Serve warm or allow to cool and refrigerate for later.

PER SERVING

Calories: 293 | Fat: 7g | Protein: 14g | Sodium: 1,512mg | Fiber: 12g | Carbohydrates: 44g | Sugar: 11g

Creamy Potato Soup

Prep time: 5 minutes | Cook time: 35 minutes| Serves 5

- 2 medium russet potatoes
- 1½ cups low-sodium chicken broth
- 1½ cups whole milk
- ½ cup sour cream
- ½ cup shredded Cheddar cheese
- 6 tablespoons chopped chives
- 1 teaspoon salt
- 1 teaspoon ground black pepper
- 3 slices bacon, cooked and crumbled

1. Preheat oven to 400°F.
2. Place potatoes on a baking sheet and bake 1 hour. Cool 10 minutes, then cut potatoes in half. Scoop the flesh from each half and roughly dice. Set aside.
3. Place cauliflower in a steamer basket. In a medium saucepan, bring 1" of water to a boil. Place steamer basket in saucepan, cover, and reduce heat to medium-low. Steam cauliflower for 5 minutes.
4. Remove from heat, then transfer soup to a blender and process until smooth (or use a handheld blender).
5. Return soup to pot and place over low heat and stir in sour cream, cheese, chives, salt, and pepper. Simmer 10 minutes, stirring frequently.
6. Top with bacon before serving.

PER SERVING

Calories: 186 | Fat: 9 g | Sodium: 609mg | Carbohydrates: 19g | Fiber: 3 g | Sugar: 3g | Protein: 7 g

Sweet Potato Soup

Prep time: 5 minutes | Cook time: 35 minutes| Serves 4

- 6 large sweet potatoes, peeled and chopped
- 1 large onion, peeled and chopped
- 3 stalks celery, chopped
- 2 teaspoons poultry seasoning
- 4 cups low-sodium chicken broth
- 2 cups milk

1. Add sweet potatoes, onion, celery, and poultry seasoning to a large pot. Add broth and top off with water until vegetables are just covered.
2. Bring to a boil over high heat. Reduce heat to medium-low and simmer 10–15 minutes until vegetables are tender.
3. Remove from heat, then transfer soup to a blender and process until smooth (or use a handheld blender). Return soup to pot and stir in milk. Heat over medium-low heat for 5 minutes. Serve hot.

PER SERVING

Calories: 178| Fat: 3g | Sodium: 121mg | Carbohydrates:29g | Fiber: 4g| Sugar: 12 g | Protein: 8g

Garlic Cheddar Cauliflower Soup

Prep time: 5 minutes | Cook time: 35 minutes| Serves 2

- 2 tablespoons olive oil
- 1 small yellow onion, peeled and chopped
- 2 cloves garlic, peeled and minced
- 1 medium head cauliflower, cored, outer leaves removed, and chopped
- 4 cups low-sodium chicken broth
- ½ cup shredded sharp Cheddar cheese
- ¼ cup grated Parmesan cheese

1. Heat oil in a large saucepan over medium heat. Sauté onion and garlic 5 minutes.
2. Add cauliflower and broth. Increase heat to high and bring to a boil.
3. Reduce heat to medium-low and simmer 20 minutes until cauliflower is soft.
4. Remove from heat, then transfer soup to a blender and process until smooth (or use a handheld blender).
5. Return soup to pot, stir in Cheddar and Parmesan, and heat, stirring constantly, over medium heat 5 minutes until cheeses melt. Serve hot.

PER SERVING

Calories: 351| Fat: 23g | Sodium: 485mg | Carbohydrates:18g | Fiber: 7g| Sugar: 8g | Protein: 18g

Cheese and Turkey Sandwiches

Prep time: 10 minutes | Cook time: 4 minutes | Serves 2

- 1 tablespoon olive oil
- 4 ounces (113 g) sliced turkey
- 2 slices reduced-fat Swiss cheese
- ½ cup sauerkraut, drained
- ¼ cup fat-free Thousand Island dressing
- 4 slices rye bread

1. Heat oil in a nonstick skillet over medium heat.
2. While pan heats, evenly divide turkey, cheese, sauerkraut, and dressing between the slices of rye bread, stacking two with toppings, then topping with the remaining two slices.
3. Cook sandwich in skillet 3–4 minutes per side, until bread is toasted and warm, then serve.

PER SERVING

Calories: 403 | Fat: 15 g | Protein: 23 g | Sodium: 1,502mg | Fiber: 6 g | Carbohydrates: 43g | Sugar: 9g

Broccoli and "Cheese" Soup

Prep time: 5 minutes | Cook time: 25 minutes| Serves 4

- 1 teaspoon olive oil
- 1 medium yellow onion, peeled and chopped
- 2 teaspoons minced garlic
- 3 cups low-sodium chicken broth
- 1 cup full-fat coconut milk
- 5 cups roughly chopped broccoli florets
- ⅓ cup nutritional yeast
- ¼ teaspoon salt

1. Heat oil in a large pot over medium heat. Add onion and garlic and sauté for 3–4 minutes until softened.
2. Add chicken broth, coconut milk, broccoli, nutritional yeast, and salt. Stir to combine.
3. Reduce heat to medium-low and simmer for 12–15 minutes until broccoli is tender.
4. Remove from heat, then transfer soup to a blender and process until smooth or until desired consistency is reached (or use a handheld blender). Serve immediately.

PER SERVING

Calories: 208| Fat: 17g | Sodium: 178mg| Carbohydrates:11g | Fiber: 1g| Sugar: 6g | Protein: 3g

Instant Pot® Chicken and White Bean Soup

Prep time: 5 minutes | Cook time: 35 minutes| Serves 6

- 1 ½ pounds boneless, skinless chicken breasts
- 3 cups low-sodium chicken broth, divided
- 2 tablespoons salted butter
- 1 tablespoon minced garlic
- 1 (4.5-ounce) can chopped green chilies, drained
- 1 tablespoon ground cumin
- 1 teaspoon dried oregano
- 1 teaspoon salt
- ½ teaspoon ground black pepper
- 2 (15-ounce) cans white beans, drained and rinsed
- ¼ cup chopped fresh cilantro

1. Place chicken, 2 cups broth, butter, onion, garlic, chilies, cumin, oregano, salt, and pepper in an Instant Pot®.
2. Close lid, set steam release to Sealing, press the Manual button, and set time to 19 minutes. When the timer beeps, quick-release the pressure until the float valve drops and open the lid.
3. Transfer chicken to a plate and cool 5 minutes. Shred chicken with two forks and return it to the Instant Pot®. Stir in beans and the remaining 1 cup broth. Let soup stand on the Keep Warm setting for 5 minutes.
4. Garnish soup with fresh cilantro before serving.

PER SERVING

Calories: 270| Fat: 5g | Sodium: 820mg |
Carbohydrates: 25g| Fiber: 5g| Sugar: 1g | Protein: 32g

Broiled Tomato Sandwiches

Prep time: 10 minutes | Cook time: 5 minutes | Serves 5

- 2 tablespoons olive oil
- 2 tablespoons balsamic vinegar
- 1 large tomato, sliced
- 3 tablespoons mayonnaise
- ½ teaspoon dried parsley
- ¼ teaspoon ground black pepper
- 4 slices whole-grain bread

1. Preheat broiler.
2. In a small bowl, whisk oil and vinegar together. Add tomato, cover, and set aside to marinate for 30–60 minutes.
3. In a separate small bowl, mix mayonnaise, parsley, oregano, pepper, and cheese.
4. Place bread slices on a baking sheet and spread with mayonnaise mixture. Top 2 of the slices with marinated tomatoes. Place remaining 2 bread slices on top of tomatoes, mayonnaise side down.
5. Broil 5 minutes or until bread is toasted and golden brown. Serve immediately.

PER SERVING

Calories: 466 | Fat: 31 g | Protein: 8 g | Sodium: 287mg |
Fiber: 5 g | Carbohydrates: 40g | Sugar: 9 g

Slow Cooker Black Bean Soup

Prep time: 5 minutes | Cook time: 4 hour 15 minutes| Serves 6

- 2 tablespoons olive oil
- 2 medium carrots, peeled and chopped
- 2 stalks celery, chopped
- 1 medium onion, peeled and chopped
- ¼ cup tomato paste
- 3 cloves garlic, peeled and minced
- 1 ½ teaspoons ground cumin
- 3 (15-ounce) cans black beans, drained and rinsed
- 1 cup frozen or canned corn
- 3 cups vegetable broth

1. Heat oil in a medium skillet over medium-high heat.
2. Add carrots, celery, and onion to the pan and sauté 5 minutes until slightly softened.
3. Stir in tomato paste, garlic, and cumin and continue to cook 2 minutes, stirring frequently.
4. Transfer mixture to a 4- to 6-quart slow cooker. Stir in beans, corn, and broth. Cook on high for 4 hours.
5. Serve warm or allow to cool and refrigerate for up to 5 days.

PER SERVING

Calories: 392| Fat: 6g | Sodium: 102mg |
Carbohydrates:66g | Fiber: 2g| Sugar: 6g | Protein: 18g

Turkey Pumpkin Chili

Prep time: 5 minutes | Cook time: 35 minutes| Serves 4

- 1 tablespoon olive oil
- 1 pound ground turkey
- 1 medium yellow onion, peeled and diced
- 1 tablespoon minced garlic
- 2 tablespoons chili powder
- 1 tablespoon ground cumin
- 1 teaspoon paprika
- ½ teaspoon pumpkin pie spice
- 1 cup canned crushed tomatoes
- 1 cup canned pumpkin purée
- 1 ½ cups water
- 1 teaspoon salt

1. Heat oil in a large skillet over medium-high heat. Add ground turkey, onion, and garlic and sauté for about 7–8 minutes, or until turkey is no longer pink.
2. Add chili powder, cumin, paprika, pumpkin pie spice, tomatoes, pumpkin, water, and salt. Bring to a boil.
3. Reduce heat to low and simmer 20 minutes.
4. Ladle into four bowls and serve.

PER SERVING

Calories: 253| Fat: 12g | Sodium: 785mg|
Carbohydrates:14g | Fiber:4 g | Sugar: 7g | Protein: 24g

Spicy Ranch Chili

Prep time: 5 minutes | Cook time: 35 minutes| Serves 6

- 2 (15-ounce) cans chili beans
- 2 tablespoons olive oil
- 1 small yellow onion, peeled and diced
- 2 medium red bell peppers, seeded and diced
- 2 tablespoons ranch seasoning mix
- 2 teaspoons chili powder
- 1 (28-ounce) can diced tomatoes with juice
- 2 tablespoons sriracha sauce

1. Drain and rinse 1 can of chili beans. Set aside.
2. In a large saucepan, heat oil over medium-high heat. Add onion and peppers and sauté until softened, about 6–8 minutes.
3. Stir in ranch seasoning and chili powder. Add drained and undrained beans, tomatoes, and sriracha and bring to a boil.
4. Reduce heat to medium-low. Simmer for 15–20 minutes until thickened. Serve immediately.

PER SERVING

Calories: 154| Fat: 4g | Sodium:391mg |
Carbohydrates:20g | Fiber: 6g| Sugar: 6g | Protein: 7g

Creamy Pumpkin Soup

Prep time: 5 minutes | Cook time: 18 minutes| Serves 4

- 4 cups low-sodium chicken broth
- 1 (15-ounce) can pumpkin purée
- 2 cups full-fat coconut milk
- ½ teaspoon salt
- ½ teaspoon ground cinnamon
- ¼ teaspoon ground ginger
- ¼ teaspoon ground nutmeg

1. Place all ingredients in a large saucepan and stir to combine.
2. Bring to a boil over high heat. Reduce heat to low, cover, and simmer for 12–15 minutes until fully warmed.
3. Serve hot.

PER SERVING

Calories: 363| Fat: 30g | Sodium:340mg |
Carbohydrates:21g | Fiber: 2g| Sugar: 9g | Protein: 1g

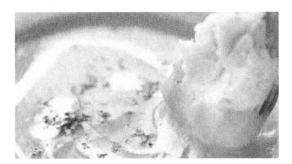

Turkey Reuben Sandwiches

Prep time: 5 minutes | Cook time: 8 minutes| Serves 2

- 1 tablespoon olive oil
- 4 slices rye bread
- 4 ounces sliced turkey breast
- 2 slices Swiss cheese
- ½ cup sauerkraut, drained
- ¼ cup Thousand Island dressing

1. Heat oil in a medium skillet over medium heat.
2. Place 2 slices of bread on a flat surface. Top each with turkey, cheese, sauerkraut, and dressing. Top with the remaining slices of bread.
3. Cook sandwiches in the skillet 3–4 minutes per side until bread is toasted. Serve warm.

PER SERVING

Calories:577 | Fat: 28g | Sodium: 954mg|
Carbohydrates:59g | Fiber: 2g| Sugar: 8g | Protein: 22g

Smashed Chickpea and Avocado Sandwiches

Prep time: 5 minutes | Cook time: 5 minutes| Serves 2

- 1 (15-ounce) can chickpeas, drained, rinsed, and dried
- 1 large ripe avocado, peeled and pitted
- ¼ cup chopped fresh cilantro
- 2 tablespoons lime juice
- ⅛ teaspoon salt
- ⅛ teaspoon ground black pepper
- 4 (1-ounce) slices multigrain bread

1. Using a fork or potato masher, mash chickpeas and avocado together in a medium bowl.
2. Stir in cilantro, lime juice, salt, and pepper.
3. Spread the chickpea mixture on 2 slices of bread. Top with the remaining slices of bread. Cut each sandwich in half and serve immediately.

PER SERVING

Calories: 442| Fat: 14g | Sodium: 829mg|
Carbohydrates:64g | Fiber: 22g| Sugar: 2g | Protein: 19g

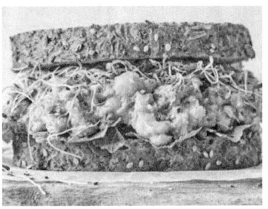

Turkey and Spinach Focaccia Sandwiches

Prep time: 5 minutes | Cook time: 5 minutes| Serves 2

- 2 tablespoons mayonnaise
- 2 tablespoons chopped fresh basil
- 2 tablespoons diced sun-dried tomatoes
- ¼ teaspoon crushed red pepper
- 4 (1-ounce) slices focaccia bread
- 8 ounces sliced turkey breast
- 1 cup baby spinach

1. In a small bowl, mix mayonnaise, basil, tomatoes, and crushed red pepper.
2. Place 2 slices bread on a flat surface. Spread each with mayonnaise mixture, then top with turkey and spinach. Cover with the remaining 2 slices bread. Cut in half and serve.

PER SERVING

Calories: 539| Fat: 25g | Sodium:1,042mg | Carbohydrates:58g | Fiber: 3g| Sugar:4 g | Protein: 20g

Apple and Cheddar Waffle Sandwich

Prep time: 5 minutes | Cook time: 8 minutes| Serves 1

- 2 frozen whole-grain waffles
- 2 teaspoons honey mustard
- 1 (1-ounce) slice Cheddar cheese
- ½ small apple, cored and thinly sliced

1. Toast waffles in a toaster oven for 2 minutes.
2. Spread 1 teaspoon honey mustard on each waffle.
3. Top 1 waffle with Cheddar cheese and the other with apple slices.
4. Return waffles to the toaster oven and toast for another 2 minutes or until cheese is melted and bubbly.
5. Carefully remove waffles from toaster oven. Press waffles together with Cheddar and apples on the inside. Serve immediately.

PER SERVING

Calories: 278| Fat: 10g | Sodium: 691mg| Carbohydrates:37g | Fiber: 4g | Sugar: 9g | Protein: 11g

The Red Onion Sandwich

Prep time: 5 minutes | Cook time: 5 minutes| Serves 1

- 1 ½ tablespoons mayonnaise
- 1 tablespoon finely chopped sun-dried tomatoes, drained
- 2 (1-ounce) slices whole-grain bread
- 3 ounces sliced turkey breast
- 1 (1-ounce) slice sharp Cheddar cheese
- 2 slices thick-cut bacon, cooked
- ⅓ medium Granny Smith apple, cored and thinly sliced
- 2 thin slices red onion

1. In a small bowl, combine mayonnaise and sun-dried tomatoes. Use the back of a spoon to muddle and break up sun-dried tomatoes as much as possible.
2. Spread mayonnaise mixture on 1 bread slice. Top with turkey, cheese, bacon, apple, and onion.
3. Place the other bread slice on top and toast for 1–2 minutes in a toaster oven until bread is lightly browned and cheese is fully melted.
4. Slice in half and serve immediately.

PER SERVING

Calories:611 | Fat: 38g | Sodium: 1,083mg| Carbohydrates:34g | Fiber: 4g| Sugar: 11g | Protein: 35g

Turkey and Cheese Pressed Sandwiches with Raspberry Jam

Prep time: 5 minutes | Cook time: 5 minutes| Serves 2

- 2 teaspoons raspberry jam
- 2 (.75-ounce) wedges creamy Swiss spreadable cheese
- 4 (1-ounce) slices multigrain bread, toasted
- 6 ounces sliced turkey breast
- 1 cup coarsely chopped baby spinach

1. In a small bowl, combine jam and cheese.
2. Spread half of the cheese mixture on 2 slices of toast. Top each with half of turkey and spinach. Cover each sandwich with the remaining slices of toast. Cut sandwiches in half and serve immediately.

PER SERVING

Calories: 347| Fat: 9g | Sodium:987mg | Carbohydrates:44g | Fiber: 9g| Sugar: 10g | Protein: 20g

Buffalo Chicken Mini Wraps

Prep time: 5 minutes | Cook time:2 hours 35 minutes| Serves 15

- 3 (6-ounce) boneless, skinless chicken breasts, cut into ½" cubes
- ¾ cup Frank's RedHot Original Cayenne Pepper Sauce, divided
- 15 (4") corn tortillas
- 1 medium avocado, peeled, pitted, and diced
- ½ cup ranch dressing

1. Place chicken in a large bowl or zip-top plastic bag. Pour ½ cup hot sauce over chicken, toss to coat, and refrigerate 2 hours.
2. Spray a large skillet with nonstick cooking spray and heat over medium heat. Add marinated chicken to pan and sauté 10–12 minutes until fully cooked.
3. Remove from heat and add remaining ¼ cup hot sauce to chicken. Toss to coat, then set aside to cool for 5 minutes.
4. Place tortillas on a flat surface. Divide chicken mixture among tortillas and top with avocado. Drizzle with dressing.
5. Roll each filled tortilla into a cylinder. Serve warm or refrigerate for up to 3 days.

PER SERVING

Calories: 142| Fat: 7g | Sodium:543mg | Carbohydrates:11g | Fiber: 2g| Sugar: 1g | Protein: 9g

Fig and Bacon Grilled Cheese Panini

Prep time: 5 minutes | Cook time: 15 minutes| Serves 2

- 4 (1-ounce) slices whole-wheat bread
- 4 tablespoons fig spread
- 2 (1-ounce) slices Cheddar cheese
- 4 slices bacon, cooked

1. Preheat a panini press or grill pan.
2. Spread each slice of bread with 1 tablespoon fig spread.
3. Place 1 cheese slice and 2 bacon slices on each of 2 slices of bread. Top with remaining bread slices.
4. Grill sandwiches in the panini press or on the grill pan until cheese has melted and bread is toasted and golden, about 8 minutes.
5. Slice each sandwich in half and serve immediately.

PER SERVING

Calories:422 | Fat: 21g | Sodium:920mg |
Carbohydrates:39g | Fiber: 4g| Sugar: 21g | Protein: 20g

Cilantro Chicken and Avocado Burritos

Prep time: 5 minutes | Cook time: 5 minutes| Serves 4

- 4 (8") flour tortillas
- 1 pound boneless, skinless chicken breasts, cooked and shredded
- 1 medium avocado, peeled, pitted, and diced
- 1 cup shredded Mexican-blend cheese
- 1 cup salsa verde
- ½ cup sour cream
- 4 tablespoons chopped fresh cilantro

1. Place tortillas on a work surface.
2. Equally distribute chicken, avocado, cheese, salsa, sour cream, and cilantro among tortillas.
3. Roll up tortillas and serve.

PER SERVING

Calories:425 | Fat: 22g | Sodium: 499mg|
Carbohydrates:20g | Fiber: 2g| Sugar: 0g | Protein: 32g

Open-Faced BLATs

Prep time: 5 minutes | Cook time: 15 minutes| Serves 4

- 12 slices center-cut bacon
- 1 medium avocado, pitted and peeled
- ¼ teaspoon salt
- ¼ teaspoon ground black pepper
- 4 (1-ounce) slices whole-grain bread, toasted
- 4 leaves romaine lettuce
- 1 medium tomato, cut into 8 slices

1. Cook bacon in a large skillet over medium heat until crisp, 8–10 minutes. Transfer to a paper towel-lined plate and set aside.
2. Mash avocado in a medium bowl with salt and pepper.
3. Spread avocado mixture on each slice of toast.
4. Top each with 3 pieces of bacon, 1 lettuce leaf, and 2 tomato slices. Serve immediately.

PER SERVING

Calories: 205| Fat: 13g | Sodium:592mg |
Carbohydrates: 14g| Fiber: 4g| Sugar: 6g | Protein: 8g

Turkey Kale Wraps

Prep time: 5 minutes | Cook time: 5 minutes| Serves 4

- 4 large leaves lacinato kale
- ⅔ cup garlic hummus
- 8 ounces sliced turkey breast
- ½ small cucumber, thinly sliced

1. Place kale leaves on a flat surface.
2. Spread hummus on kale and top with turkey and cucumber.
3. Roll leaves into cylinders and serve immediately.

PER SERVING

Calories:137 | Fat: 5g | Sodium:690mg |
Carbohydrates:11g | Fiber: 2g| Sugar: 2g | Protein: 12g

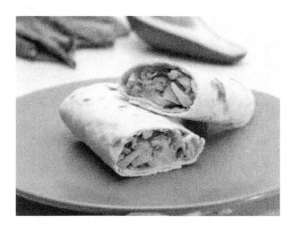

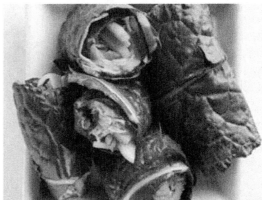

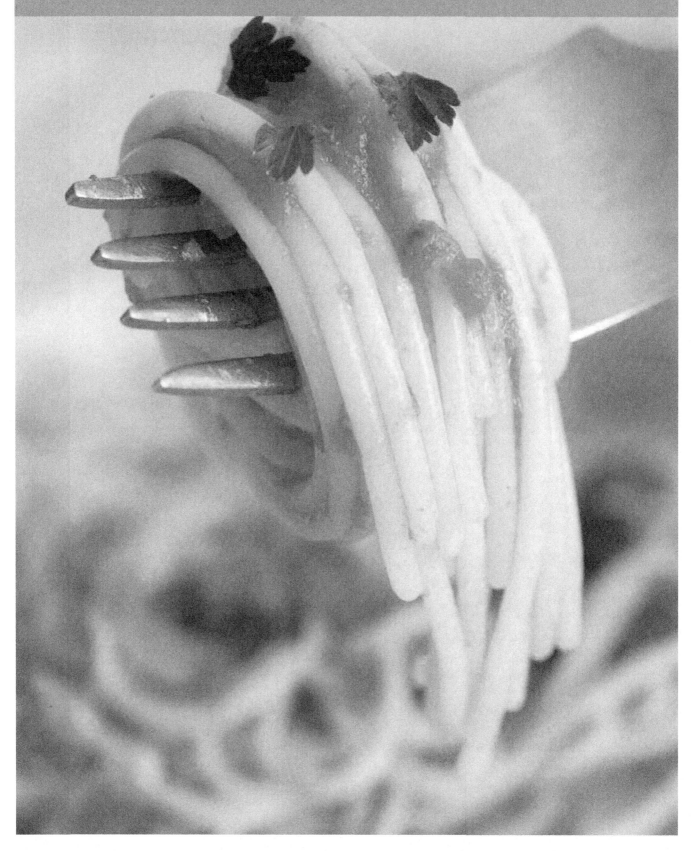

Carrot Shredded Chicken with Ramen

Prep time: 10 minutes | Cook time: 5 minutes | Serves 4

- 3 cups water
- 1 (3-ounce) package chicken-flavored ramen noodles, with seasoning package
- 2 cups cooked, shredded chicken breast
- 2 bok choy leaves, sliced into strips
- 1 medium carrot, sliced and peeled
- 1 teaspoon sesame oil

1. Bring water to a boil in a large pot.
2. Add all other ingredients and simmer 3–5 minutes before serving.

PER SERVING

Calories: 225 | Fat: 7 g | Protein: 24 g | Sodium: 476 mg | Fiber: 1 g | Carbohydrates: 14 g | Sugar: 1 g

Macaroni and Cheese with Chicken

Prep time: 10 minutes | Cook time: 0 minute | Serves 2

- 2 cups macaroni
- 1 tablespoon butter
- 1/2 cup fat-free shredded Cheddar cheese
- 6 ounces grilled chicken, cut into strips
- 2 tablespoons Frank's Red Hot Original Cayenne Pepper Sauce
- 1/2 cup blue cheese crumbles

1. Cook pasta according to package directions, drain, and return to pot.
2. Stir in butter and Cheddar cheese until cheese begins to melt.
3. Top with grilled chicken, drizzle with hot sauce, add blue cheese, and serve.

PER SERVING

Calories: 750 | Fat: 25 g | Protein: 48 g | Sodium: 612 mg | Fiber: 4 g | Carbohydrates: 81 g | Sugar: 3 g

Cheese, Onion and Tomato Shrimp Penne

Prep time: 10 minutes | Cook time: 20 minutes | Serves 4

- 1 (16-ounce (454g)) package whole-grain penne
- 2 tablespoons olive oil
- 1/4 cup chopped red onion
- 1 tablespoon chopped garlic
- 1/4 cup white wine
- 2 (12-ounce (340)) cans diced tomatoes
- 1 pound shrimp, peeled and deveined
- 1 cup grated Parmesan cheese

1. Cook pasta according to package directions and set aside.
2. Heat oil in a medium nonstick skillet over medium-high heat. Add onion and garlic, cooking about 5 minutes until onion becomes tender.
3. Add wine and tomatoes and cook 10 more minutes, stirring frequently.
4. Add shrimp to sauce and cook an additional 5 minutes. Toss shrimp with pasta and serve with Parmesan sprinkled on top.

PER SERVING

Calories: 658 | Fat: 18 g | Protein: 37 g | Sodium: 1,196 mg | Fiber: 12 g | Carbohydrates: 90 g | Sugar: 7 g

Macaroni and Tuna Salad with Feta

Prep time: 10 minutes | Cook time: 0 minute | Serves 2

- 1 cup whole-grain dry macaroni
- 1 (5-ounce (425g)) can tuna, drained and rinsed
- 1/3 cup feta cheese
- 3 cherry tomatoes
- 1 tablespoon olive oil
- 1/4 teaspoon salt
- 1/4 teaspoon freshly ground black pepper

1. Cook pasta according to package directions and drain.
2. Add tuna and feta cheese to hot pasta, stirring until cheese begins to melt.
3. Add remaining ingredients, mix well, and serve.

PER SERVING

Calories: 467 | Fat: 20 g | Protein: 32 g | Sodium: 816 mg | Fiber: 5.5 g | Carbohydrates: 43 g | Sugar: 3 g

Spicy Buffalo Macaroni and Cheese

Prep time: 5 minutes | Cook time: 15 minutes | Serves 2

- 2 cups elbow macaroni
- 1 tablespoon salted butter
- 1/2 cup fat-free shredded Cheddar cheese
- 6 ounces grilled chicken, cut into strips
- 2 tablespoons Frank's RedHot Original Cayenne Pepper Sauce
- 1/2 cup crumbled blue cheese

1. Fill a large pot with water and bring to a boil over high heat. Add macaroni and cook for 9 minutes. Drain and return to pot.
2. Stir in butter and Cheddar cheese until melted.
3. Top with chicken, pepper sauce, and blue cheese. Serve hot.

PER SERVING

Calories:595 | Fat: 29g | Sodium:1,435mg | Carbohydrates:40g | Fiber: 4g | Sugar: 2g | Protein: 44g

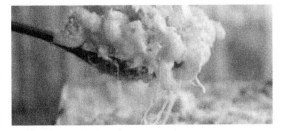

Parmesan Cheese and High-Protein Spaghetti

Prep time: 5 minutes | Cook time: 0 minute | Serves 2

- 2 cups dry whole-wheat spaghetti
- 8 ounces (227g) ground turkey, browned
- 1 cup spaghetti sauce
- 2 tablespoons grated Parmesan cheese

1. Cook pasta according to package directions and drain.
2. Add turkey and sauce to pasta, mixing well.
3. Sprinkle with grated Parmesan and serve.

PER SERVING

Calories: 601 | Fat: 14 g | Protein: 39 g | Sodium: 758 mg | Fiber: 12 g | Carbohydrates: 87 g | Sugar: 8 g

Chicken and Pesto Farfalle

Prep time: 5 minutes | Cook time: 15 minutes| Serves 4

- 8 ounces dried farfalle
- 1 cup frozen chopped green beans
- ½ cup reduced-fat pesto sauce
- 2 cups grilled chicken, cut into bite-sized pieces
- ½ cup crumbled feta or goat cheese

1. Fill a large pot with water and bring to a boil over high heat. Add pasta and cook for 11 minutes. Drain pasta, reserving ½ cup pasta cooking water.
2. Place green beans in a small skillet with enough water to cover them. Cover skillet and heat over medium heat for 5 minutes; drain.
3. Combine pasta, pesto, reserved water, chicken, green beans, and cheese in a large bowl and stir to combine. Serve hot or cold.

PER SERVING

Calories: 339| Fat: 10g | Sodium: 611mg| Carbohydrates: 25g| Fiber: 2g| Sugar: 3g | Protein: 37g

High-Protein Italian Pasta Bake

Prep time: 5 minutes | Cook time: 25 minutes| Serves 4

- 4 ounces chickpea penne pasta
- 1 pound 90% lean ground beef
- 1 (16-ounce) bag frozen pepper and onion strips, thawed
- 2 tablespoons Italian seasoning
- 1 cup marinara sauce
- 1 large egg
- 1 cup shredded mozzarella cheese

1. Preheat oven to 350°F.
2. Fill a large pot with water and bring to a boil over high heat. Add pasta and cook for 6 minutes. Drain and transfer to a large bowl.
3. Meanwhile, in a large skillet over medium-high heat, cook ground beef, breaking it up with a wooden spoon while it cooks. Sauté for 7–8

minutes until no longer pink. Add pepper and onion strips and Italian seasoning to the skillet and sauté 2 minutes.
4. Transfer ground beef mixture to the bowl with pasta. Add marinara sauce and egg. Mix ingredients well.
5. Pour ingredients into a 9" × 13" baking dish and top with cheese.
6. Bake for 10 minutes until cheese is melted. Serve immediately.

PER SERVING

Calories:438 | Fat: 21g | Sodium:348mg | Carbohydrates:24g | Fiber: 6g| Sugar: 5g | Protein: 40g

Garlicky Traditional Shrimp Scampi

Prep time: 10 minutes | Cook time: 4 minutes | Serves 4

- 1 cup dry orzo
- ½ teaspoon salt
- 2 tablespoons chopped parsley
- 4 tablespoons butter, divided
- 1½ pounds jumbo shrimp, peeled and deveined
- 1 clove garlic, minced

1. Cook orzo according to package directions. Stir in salt and parsley and set aside.
2. In a medium skillet, heat 2 tablespoons butter over medium-high heat. Sauté shrimp 2–3 minutes or until nearly cooked through and then set aside.
3. Combine remaining 2 tablespoons butter and garlic in pan and cook 30 seconds before returning shrimp to the pan.
4. Mix shrimp and garlic butter well and serve with orzo.

PER SERVING

Calories: 249 | Fat: 13 g | Protein: 12 g | Sodium: 614 mg | Fiber: 1 g | Carbohydrates: 22 g | Sugar: 1 g

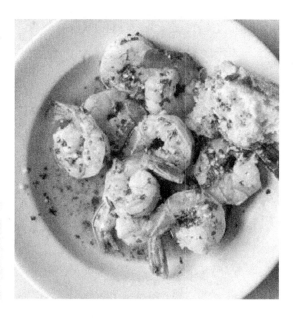

Mediterranean Shrimp Penne

Prep time: 5 minutes | Cook time: 35 minutes| Serves 4

- 12 ounces whole-grain penne
- 2 tablespoons olive oil
- ¼ cup chopped red onion
- 1 tablespoon chopped garlic
- ¼ cup white wine
- 2 (14.5-ounce) cans diced tomatoes
- 1 pound large shrimp, peeled and deveined
- ½ cup grated Parmesan cheese

1. Fill a large pot with water and bring to a boil over high heat. Add pasta and cook for 13 minutes. Drain and keep warm.
2. Heat oil in a medium nonstick skillet over medium-high heat. Add onion and garlic and sauté about 5 minutes until tender.
3. Add wine and tomatoes and cook 10 more minutes, stirring frequently. Add shrimp to sauce and cook an additional 5 minutes.
4. Toss shrimp with pasta and serve with Parmesan sprinkled on top.

PER SERVING

Calories: 547| Fat: 14g | Sodium:590mg | Carbohydrates:69g | Fiber: 13g| Sugar: 9g | Protein: 43g

Light Fettuccine Alfredo

Prep time: 5 minutes | Cook time: 35 minutes| Serves 4

- 8 ounces fettuccine
- 1 cup nonfat milk
- 6 (.75-ounce) wedges creamy mozzarella spreadable cheese
- 1 teaspoon garlic powder
- 1½ tablespoons grated Parmesan cheese
- 1 tablespoon salted butter or ghee
- ⅛ teaspoon salt
- ⅛ teaspoon ground black pepper

1. Fill a large pot with water and bring to a boil over high heat. Add pasta and cook for 12 minutes. Drain and place pasta in a large bowl.
2. In a medium saucepan over medium heat, combine spreadable cheese, garlic powder, Parmesan cheese, butter, salt, and pepper. Cook, stirring often, until everything is melted and the sauce is smooth, about 15 to 20 minutes.
3. Pour sauce over pasta and toss to combine. Serve immediately.

PER SERVING

Calories:785 | Fat: 30g | Sodium:1,520mg | Carbohydrates: 95g| Fiber: 4g| Sugar: 12g | Protein: 37g

Instant Pot® Chicken Pasta

Prep time: 5 minutes | Cook time: 25 minutes| Serves 6

- 1½ pounds boneless, skinless chicken thighs
- 4 organic chicken stock cubes
- 2 cups low-sodium chicken stock, divided
- 8 ounces high-protein chickpea pasta
- 1 (16-ounce) bag frozen mixed vegetables (corn, carrots, green beans, and peas), thawed

1. Place chicken, stock cubes, and 1 cup stock in an Instant Pot®. Close lid, set steam release to Sealing, press the Manual button, and set time to 10 minutes. When the timer beeps, quick-release the pressure until the float valve drops and open the lid.
2. Remove chicken from the pot. Shred with two forks and return to the pot with pasta and the remaining 1 cup stock. Be sure pasta is fully submerged in the liquid.
3. Close lid, set steam release to Sealing, press the Manual button, and set time to 5 minutes. When the timer beeps, quick-release the pressure until the float valve drops and open the lid. Stir in mixed vegetables. Serve immediately.

PER SERVING

Calories: 409| Fat:16 g | Sodium:1,211mg | Carbohydrates:33g | Fiber: 2g| Sugar: 8g | Protein: 33g

Garlic Parmesan Pasta

Prep time: 5 minutes | Cook time: 10 minutes| Serves 4

- 8 ounces angel hair pasta
- ¼ cup olive oil
- 1 tablespoon minced fresh oregano
- ¼ cup minced fresh parsley
- 3 teaspoons minced garlic
- ⅛ teaspoon crushed red pepper flakes
- ¼ teaspoon salt
- ¼ teaspoon ground black pepper
- ½ cup grated Parmesan cheese

1. Fill a large pot with water and bring to a boil over high heat. Add pasta and cook for 4 minutes. Drain and transfer to a large bowl.
2. Meanwhile, heat oil in a small saucepan over medium heat. Add oregano, parsley, garlic, red pepper, and salt. Sauté for 1 minute.
3. Remove from heat and pour over pasta. Toss gently to combine. Sprinkle with black pepper and cheese. Serve immediately.

PER SERVING

Calories:383 | Fat:18 g | Sodium:331mg | Carbohydrates: 42g| Fiber: 2g | Sugar: 2g | Protein: 12g

Artichoke Parmesan Pasta

Prep time: 5 minutes | Cook time: 10 minutes| Serves 4

- 8 ounces chickpea penne
- 1 (12-ounce) jar marinated artichoke hearts, undrained
- ¾ cup grated Parmesan cheese
- 2 cups baby spinach
- ½ teaspoon salt

1. Fill a large pot with water and bring to a boil over high heat. Add pasta and cook for 7 minutes. Drain and transfer to a large bowl.
2. Place artichoke hearts and liquid, cheese, spinach, and salt in a food processor and pulse until smooth. Pour sauce over pasta and stir to mix. Serve immediately.

PER SERVING

Calories: 353| Fat: 14g | Sodium:892mg |
Carbohydrates:36g | Fiber: 10g| Sugar: 5g | Protein: 23g

Ravioli Lasagna

Prep time: 5 minutes | Cook time: 65 minutes| Serves 8

- 1 pound pork sausage, casings removed
- 1 (26-ounce) jar pasta sauce, divided
- 2 (30-ounce) bags frozen large cheese ravioli, divided
- 1 (10-ounce) package frozen chopped spinach, thawed and drained
- 1½ cups shredded mozzarella cheese, divided
- ½ cup grated Parmesan cheese, divided

1. Preheat oven to 350°F. Spray a 9" × 13" baking dish with nonstick cooking spray.
2. Place sausage in a large skillet over medium-high heat. Sauté until no longer pink, about 8 minutes, using a wooden spoon to break up meat as it cooks. Drain excess fat from skillet.
3. Spread one-third of pasta sauce on the bottom of the prepared dish.
4. Arrange one-half of ravioli on top of sauce. Top with sausage and spinach. Layer one-third of pasta sauce, ¾ cup mozzarella, and ¼ cup Parmesan over sausage and spinach, then arrange remaining ravioli on top.
5. Cover with the remaining sauce, mozzarella, and Parmesan. Tightly cover the baking dish with foil.
6. Bake 45 minutes. Uncover and bake for an additional 12–15 minutes or until cheese is melted and lightly browned. Serve immediately.

PER SERVING

Calories: 694| Fat: 38g | Sodium: 1,635mg| Carbohydrates: 56g| Fiber: 19g| Sugar: 17g | Protein: 33g

Pumpkin Mac and "Cheese"

Prep time: 5 minutes | Cook time: 15 minutes| Serves 4

- 8 ounces elbow macaroni
- 1 cup unsweetened almond milk
- 1 teaspoon garlic powder
- ½ cup nutritional yeast
- ¼ teaspoon dried thyme
- 1½ teaspoons Dijon mustard
- 1 cup canned pumpkin purée
- 1 tablespoon maple syrup
- ¼ teaspoon salt
- ¼ teaspoon ground black pepper

1. Fill a large pot with water and bring to a boil over high heat. Add pasta and cook for 9 minutes. Drain and transfer to a large bowl.
2. Meanwhile, heat milk in a small saucepan over medium heat for 2 minutes. Add garlic powder, nutritional yeast, thyme, mustard, pumpkin, maple syrup, salt, and pepper and whisk until thoroughly combined. Reduce heat to low and cook until the sauce has thickened, about 5 minutes.
3. Pour the pumpkin sauce over the macaroni and mix well. Serve hot.

PER SERVING

Calories:257 | Fat: 3g | Sodium: 247mg|
Carbohydrates:50g | Fiber: 5g| Sugar: 7g | Protein:8 g

Buffalo Blue Chicken Pasta

Prep time: 5 minutes | Cook time: 20 minutes| Serves 4

- 8 ounces chickpea rotini pasta
- 1 teaspoon salted butter or ghee
- ½ cup diced onion
- ⅓ cup Frank's RedHot Original Cayenne Pepper Sauce
- 8 ounces Instant Pot® Shredded Chicken
- 4 ounces crumbled blue cheese

1. Fill a large pot with water and bring to a boil over high heat. Add pasta and cook for 7 minutes. Drain, transfer to a large bowl, and set aside.
2. Melt butter in a large skillet over medium heat. Sauté onion 5–7 minutes until soft and translucent. Add pasta, pepper sauce, and chicken. Mix well, then top with cheese. Serve immediately.

PER SERVING

Calories:325 | Fat: 9g | Sodium: 1,134mg|
Carbohydrates:44g | Fiber: 11g| Sugar: 3g | Protein: 19g

Cheesy Edamame Spaghetti

Prep time: 5 minutes | Cook time: 15 minutes | Serves 4

- 4 ounces brown rice spaghetti
- 1 cup unsalted roasted cashews
- ⅓ cup grated Parmesan cheese
- 1 teaspoon garlic powder
- ½ teaspoon salt
- 3 cups frozen edamame, thawed
- 2 cups finely chopped fresh parsley
- 2 teaspoons extra-virgin olive oil
- ½ teaspoon ground black pepper

1. Fill a large pot with water and bring to a boil over high heat. Add pasta and cook for 10 minutes. Drain and transfer to a large bowl.
2. Add cashews, cheese, garlic powder, and salt to a food processor. Pulse until a coarse texture is achieved. Set aside.
3. Toss pasta with edamame, parsley, oil, and pepper. Top with cashew mixture, toss to combine, and serve.

PER SERVING

Calories:568 | Fat: 30g | Sodium:1,244mg | Carbohydrates: 49g| Fiber: 17g| Sugar: 5g | Protein: 25g

Portobello Pesto Pizzas

Prep time: 5 minutes | Cook time: 25 minutes | Serves 4

- 2 teaspoons extra-virgin olive oil
- 1 small yellow onion, peeled and diced
- 1 medium Roma tomato, diced
- 2 teaspoons minced garlic
- 4 large portobello mushroom caps
- ⅛ teaspoon salt
- ⅛ teaspoon ground black pepper
- 3 tablespoons pesto
- ¼ cup crumbled feta cheese
- 1 tablespoon balsamic vinegar

1. Preheat oven to 425°F. Line a baking sheet with parchment paper.
2. In a medium skillet, heat oil over medium heat. Add onion and sauté for 5 minutes or until soft and translucent. Add tomato and garlic. Sauté for another 5 minutes, then remove from heat and set aside.
3. Place mushroom caps (stem side up) on the prepared baking sheet. Season with salt and pepper, then spread with pesto. Top with tomato mixture and sprinkle with feta cheese. Bake for 10–12 minutes.
4. Remove from oven and drizzle with vinegar. Slice into halves or quarters with a pizza cutter. Serve immediately.

PER SERVING

Calories:99 | Fat: 7g | Sodium: 545mg| Carbohydrates: 6g| Fiber: 1g| Sugar: 2g | Protein: 3g

Creamy Bacon Pistachio Pasta

Prep time: 5 minutes | Cook time: 25 minutes | Serves 4

- 8 ounces ziti
- 4 slices thick-cut bacon
- ¼ cup fat-free ricotta cheese
- ½ cup grated Parmesan cheese
- ¼ cup 1% milk
- ½ tablespoon extra-virgin olive oil
- ¼ teaspoon salt
- ¼ teaspoon ground black pepper
- ¼ cup shelled pistachios

1. Fill a large pot with water and bring to a boil over high heat. Add pasta and cook for 9 minutes. Drain and transfer to a large bowl.
2. In a medium skillet over medium heat, cook bacon for 8–10 minutes or until crisp. Drain on paper towels and chop coarsely.
3. In a small bowl, combine ricotta, Parmesan, milk, oil, salt, and pepper; blend well. Add cheese mixture to pasta and mix well.
4. Stir in bacon and pistachios. Serve immediately.

PER SERVING

Calories:394 | Fat: 14g | Sodium:716mg | Carbohydrates: 46g| Fiber: 2g| Sugar: 5g | Protein: 20g

Pesto Chicken Pizza

Prep time: 5 minutes | Cook time: 15 minutes | Serves 6

- 1 (12", 10-ounce) thin pizza crust
- ¾ cup pesto
- 1 cup chopped rotisserie chicken breast
- 6 ounces fresh mozzarella cheese, sliced
- 1 medium tomato, sliced
- ¾ cup crumbled feta cheese

1. Preheat oven to 450°F.
2. Place pizza crust on a pizza pan or baking sheet.
3. Spread pesto evenly over crust. Top with chicken, mozzarella, tomato slices, and feta.
4. Bake for 8–10 minutes until cheese is fully melted. (For a crispier crust, bake the pizza directly on the oven rack.)
5. Remove from oven and cool for 5 minutes before cutting.

PER SERVING

Calories: 430| Fat: 25g | Sodium: 878mg| Carbohydrates: 26g| Fiber: 0g| Sugar: 4g | Protein: 26g

Mini Buffalo Chicken Pizzas

Prep time: 5 minutes | Cook time: 15 minutes| Serves 4

- 4 English muffins, sliced in half
- ½ cup pizza sauce
- ½ cup Frank's RedHot Original Cayenne Pepper Sauce
- 2 teaspoons Tabasco sauce
- ½ teaspoon dried oregano
- ½ teaspoon garlic powder
- 2 cups Buffalo-Style Shredded Chicken
- 2 cups shredded mozzarella cheese
- 2 tablespoons ranch salad dressing
- 2 scallions, finely chopped

1. Preheat oven to 350°F. Place English muffin halves on a large baking sheet, cut side up.
2. In a small bowl, combine pizza sauce, pepper sauce, Tabasco sauce, oregano, and garlic powder. Spread mixture on English muffins. Top with chicken and cheese.
3. Bake for 10 minutes until the cheese is melted. Remove from oven, drizzle with dressing, top with scallions, and serve.

PER SERVING

Calories: 463| Fat: 19g | Sodium:2,034mg |
Carbohydrates:36g | Fiber: 5g| Sugar: 5g | Protein: 35g

Broccoli and Cheddar Pita Pizzas

Prep time: 5 minutes | Cook time: 15 minutes| Serves 2

- 1 teaspoon olive oil
- ¾ cup frozen broccoli florets, chopped
- ⅛ teaspoon salt
- 2 (8") whole-wheat pitas
- ½ cup hummus
- 2 (1-ounce) slices Cheddar cheese

1. Preheat oven to 375°F. Line a baking sheet with parchment paper.
2. In a small skillet, heat oil over medium-high heat. Sauté broccoli until thawed. Season with salt.
3. Place pitas on the prepared baking sheet. Spread hummus over pitas in a thick layer and top with broccoli and a slice of cheese.
4. Bake for 8–10 minutes until cheese is melted and the pita is lightly toasted. Cool slightly and slice into quarters before serving.

PER SERVING

Calories:319 | Fat: 19g | Sodium: 634mg|
Carbohydrates:25g | Fiber: 7g| Sugar: 4g | Protein: 11g

Low-Carb Eggplant Pizzas

Prep time: 5 minutes | Cook time: 15 minutes| Serves 4

- 1 large eggplant, cut into ½" slices
- ¼ cup extra-virgin olive oil
- ¼ teaspoon salt
- ¼ teaspoon ground black pepper
- ¾ cup tomato sauce
- ½ teaspoon Italian seasoning
- 4 ounces part-skim mozzarella cheese, thinly sliced
- 2 tablespoons minced fresh basil

1. Preheat broiler and line a baking sheet with parchment paper.
2. Brush each side of eggplant slices with oil and season with salt and pepper.
3. Heat a large nonstick skillet over medium heat. Cook eggplant slices in batches until tender and lightly browned, about 3–5 minutes per side.
4. Transfer eggplant slices to the prepared baking sheet and top each with tomato sauce, Italian seasoning, and cheese.
5. Broil for 3–5 minutes until cheese is melted and lightly browned.
6. Top with basil and serve.

PER SERVING

Calories: 248| Fat: 17g | Sodium:401mg |
Carbohydrates: 12g| Fiber: 5g| Sugar: 6g | Protein: 11g

Spinach, Sausage, and Provolone Pizza

Prep time: 5 minutes | Cook time: 25 minutes| Serves 6

- 1 tablespoon olive oil
- 8 ounces Italian sausage, casings removed
- 3 cups baby spinach
- ¼ teaspoon salt
- ⅛ teaspoon ground black pepper
- 1 pound pizza dough
- 4 ounces sharp provolone cheese, thinly sliced

1. Preheat oven to 425°F. Spray a baking sheet with nonstick cooking spray.
2. Heat oil in a large skillet over medium-high heat. Add sausage and cook, breaking it up with a spoon, until no longer pink, 4–5 minutes. Add spinach, salt, and pepper. Toss 1 minute until spinach is wilted.
3. Spread dough on the prepared baking sheet. Top with cheese, then sausage mixture.
4. Bake until crust is crisp and cheese has melted, 12–15 minutes.
5. Remove from oven. Cool for 5 minutes before slicing and serving.

PER SERVING

Calories:225 | Fat: 6g | Sodium:202mg |
Carbohydrates:34g | Fiber: 1g| Sugar: 0g | Protein: 9g

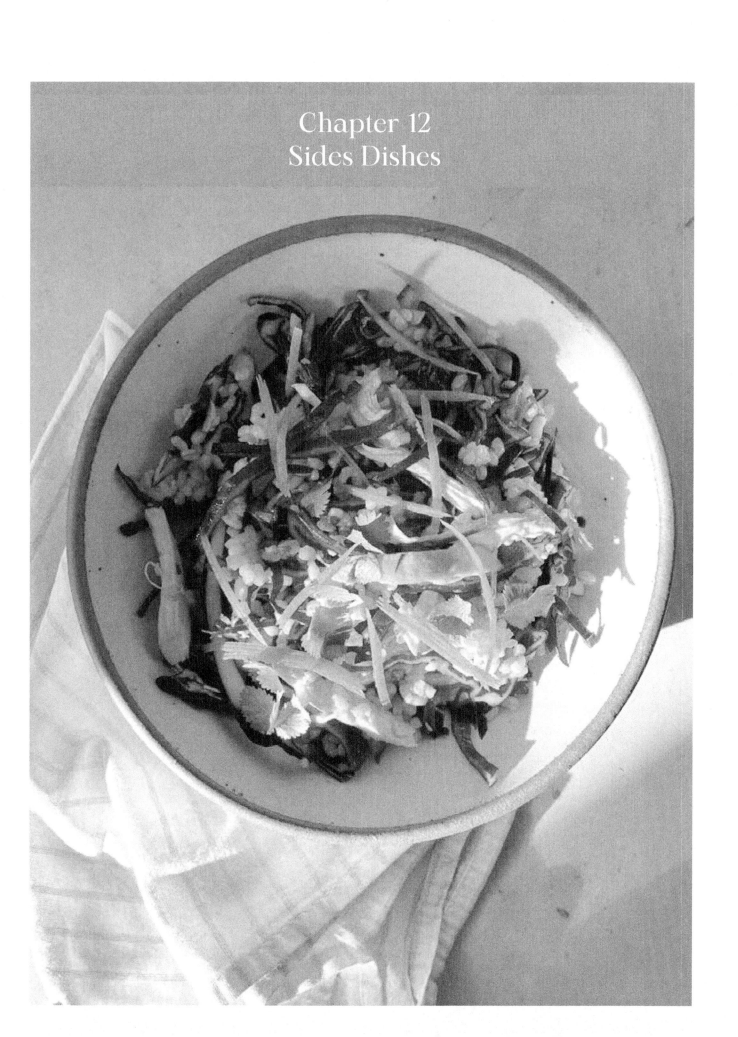

Chapter 12
Sides Dishes

Garlic Parmesan Fries

Prep time: 10 minutes | Cook time: 20 minutes | Serves 2

- 1 teaspoon olive oil
- 1 clove garlic, peeled and crushed
- 1 large potato, cut into sticks
- ½ teaspoon salt
- 1 tablespoon grated Parmesan cheese
- 1 tablespoon chopped parsley

1. Preheat oven to 425°F (220°C).
2. In a medium bowl, combine oil and garlic and toss potato sticks in mixture, coating well.
3. Arrange fries on a baking sheet, spreading evenly, and sprinkle with salt. Bake for 10 minutes per side.
4. Remove from the oven, top with Parmesan and parsley, and serve.

PER SERVING

Calories: 172g | Fat: 3 g | Protein: 4 g | Sodium: 623 mg | Fiber: 4g | Carbohydrates: 32 g | Sugar: 2 g

Limey Cilantro and Potato Rice

Prep time: 10 minutes | Cook time: 5 minutes | Serves 4

- 1 (10-ounce (283g)) bag frozen riced cauliflower, thawed
- 3 tablespoons water
- 2 tablespoons lime juice
- 2 teaspoons grated lime zest
- ½ cup chopped fresh cilantro

1. Combine cauliflower and water in a large microwave-safe bowl and microwave on high 3–5 minutes until cauliflower is soft.
2. Stir in lime juice, zest, and cilantro. Mix well and serve immediately.

PER SERVING

Calories: 16g | Fat: 0 g | Protein: 1 g | Sodium: 44 mg | Fiber: 1g | Carbohydrates: 3 g | Sugar: 0 g

Stuffed Bell Peppers

Prep time: 5 minutes | Cook time: 50 minutes| Serves 4

- 4 medium red bell peppers (600g), seeded
- 4 teaspoons (20ml) extra-virgin olive oil, divided
- 1 pound (453g) extra-lean ground beef or turkey
- 1 medium onion (94g), finely diced
- 1 large tomato (182g), chopped
- 1 to 1½ tablespoons (4 to 6g) minced fresh cilantro
- 1 to 1½ tablespoon (4 to 6g) minced fresh parsley
- 2 tablespoons (18g) pine nuts
- ¼ to ½ teaspoon (0.7 to 1.2g) ground cinnamon
- ¼ teaspoon (0.5g) ground allspice
- ¼ teaspoon (0.5g) freshly ground black pepper
- 1 teaspoon (6g) sea salt
- 1½ cups (375g) tomato sauce or marinara sauce

1. Preheat the oven to 350°F.
2. Cut the tops off the peppers and reserve for later.
3. In a large skillet over medium heat, heat 2 teaspoons of olive oil and add the peppers and tops. Lightly sauté until they soften but still retain their shape, 3 to 5 minutes. Set aside.
4. In the same pan, heat the remaining oil. Add the beef and sauté 7 to 10 minutes, then add the onions and sauté until golden brown, about 7 minutes. Add the tomato, cilantro, parsley, pine nuts, cinnamon, allspice, pepper, and salt and mix. Remove from the heat.
5. Sit the peppers upright on an 8-by-8-inch square glass ovenproof pan, and stuff them with the meat filling.
6. Put the tops on the peppers. Pour the tomato sauce into the dish.
7. Bake, uncovered, until the peppers are tender, about 30 minutes. Remove from the oven and let cool.
8. Into each of 4 airtight storage containers, place 1 stuffed pepper and seal.

PER SERVING

Calories: 322| Fat: 13g| Protein: 28g| Total Carbs: 14g| Net Carbs: 10g| Fiber: 4g| Sugar: 12g| Sodium: 1038mg

Sweet Potato Wedges

Prep time: 5 minutes | Cook time: 35 minutes | Serves 4

- 4 medium sweet potatoes, cut into thick wedges
- 2 ½ tablespoons olive oil
- ½ teaspoon paprika
- ½ teaspoon garlic powder
- 1 teaspoon salt
- ½ teaspoon ground black pepper

1. Preheat oven to 400°F (205°C).
2. Combine all ingredients in a large bowl, tossing until sweet potatoes are well coated. Arrange on a baking sheet.
3. Cook 30–35 minutes, turning halfway through, until fries reach desired level of crispness. Serve.

PER SERVING

Calories: 193g | Fat: 8g | Protein: 1 g | Sodium: 626 mg | Fiber: 1g | Carbohydrates: 31g | Sugar: 7 g

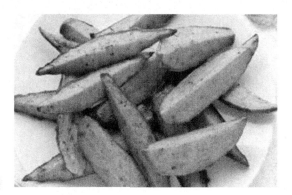

Garlicky Zucchini Fries with Cheese

Prep time: 10 minutes | Cook time: 20 minutes | Serves 4

- 1 cup dried bread crumbs
- ¼ teaspoon garlic powder
- 2 tablespoons grated Parmesan cheese
- ¼ teaspoon salt
- 3 large egg whites, beaten
- 4 medium zucchini, peeled and cut into 3" sticks

1. Preheat oven to 425°F (220°C). Line a baking sheet with parchment paper.
2. Combine bread crumbs, garlic powder, cheese, and salt in a large bowl. Place egg whites in a separate bowl.
3. Dip zucchini sticks into egg whites, toss in bread crumb mixture to coat, and arrange on the prepared baking sheet.
4. Bake 20–25 minutes or until fries begin to brown, turning halfway through.

PER SERVING

Calories: 162g | Fat: 2 g | Protein: 10 g | Sodium: 531 mg | Fiber: 4g | Carbohydrates: 27 g | Sugar: 8 g

Cabbage Slaw

Prep time: 10 minutes | Cook time: 0 minute | Serves 4

- ½ small head cabbage, shredded
- ½ medium red bell pepper, seeded and sliced
- ¼ small red onion, peeled and sliced
- 2 tablespoons olive oil
- 1 ½ tablespoons apple cider vinegar
- ¼ teaspoon salt

1. Toss all ingredients together in a large bowl.
2. Cover and refrigerate at least 1 hour before serving.

PER SERVING

Calories: 104g | Fat: 6 g | Protein: 2 g | Sodium: 169 mg | Fiber: 4g | Carbohydrates: 10 g | Sugar: 6 g

Snapper En Papillote

Prep time: 5 minutes | Cook time: 10 minutes | Serves 6

- Nonstick cooking spray
- ⅓ cup (26g) thinly sliced leeks
- ⅓ cup (29g) thinly sliced fennel
- ⅓ cup (36g) shredded carrots
- ⅓ cup (50g) thinly sliced celery
- ⅓ cup (45g) thinly sliced red bell pepper
- Sea salt
- Freshly ground black pepper
- 2¼ pounds (1kg) red snapper fillets, skin-on, cut into 6 pieces
- 3 tablespoons (42g) butter, melted
- 6 thin lemon slices (42g)

1. Preheat the oven to 450°F.

2. Cut 6 heart-shaped pieces of parchment paper large enough to contain the fish and vegetables when folded in half. Spray each piece of parchment with cooking spray and set aside.
3. In a medium bowl, toss the leeks, fennel, carrots, celery, and bell pepper. Season with salt and pepper. Divide the vegetables evenly among the pieces of prepared parchment.
4. Place one portion of red snapper on each portion of vegetables, skin-side up| brush with the melted butter, and season with salt and pepper. Place a lemon slice on top of each fillet.
5. Fold each piece of paper over the fish and vegetables, and crimp the edges to seal.
6. Place the sealed fish packets on sheet pans and bake for 8 to 10 minutes.
7. When done, the parchment paper should puff up and brown. Remove from the oven, transfer the paper packets to 6 airtight glass storage containers, open the parchment paper packets, and let cool before sealing.

PER SERVING

Calories: 310| Fat: 9g| Protein: 46g| Total Carbs: 10g| Net Carbs: 8g| Fiber: 2g| Sugar: 5g| Sodium: 171mg

Cheesy Blue Brussels Sprouts

Prep time: 5 minutes | Cook time: 20 minutes | Serves 4

- 2 tablespoons olive oil
- 1 pound Brussels sprouts, trimmed and halved
- ¼ cup Frank's Red Hot Original Cayenne Pepper Sauce
- 2 tablespoons crumbled blue cheese

1. Preheat oven to 425°F (220°C).
2. Heat oil in a large skillet over medium heat. Sauté Brussels sprouts for 4–5 minutes until softened.
3. Spread sprouts on a large baking sheet and roast for 12–15 minutes until edges start to crisp.
4. Transfer to a large bowl, toss with pepper sauce until well coated, and top with cheese before serving.

PER SERVING

Calories: 137g | Fat: 8 g | Protein: 5 g | Sodium: 656 mg | Fiber: 4g | Carbohydrates: 11 g | Sugar: 3 g

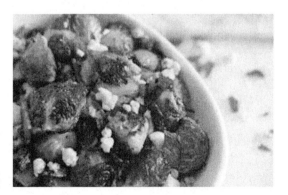

Healthy Shepherd'S Pie

Prep time: 5 minutes | Cook time: 60 minutes| Serves 8

- 8 large potatoes (1.7kg), peeled and chopped
- ¼ cup (60ml) unsweetened coconut milk
- 2 tablespoons (30ml) coconut oil
- 2½ teaspoons (15g) sea salt, divided
- ½ teaspoon (1.4g) freshly ground black pepper, divided
- Nonstick cooking spray
- 2½ pounds (1.13kg) lean ground turkey
- ½ tablespoon (0.8g) dried oregano
- ½ tablespoon (0.8g) dried parsley
- ½ tablespoon (1.6g) dried basil
- 2 cups (473ml) reduced-fat cream of mushroom soup
- 1 cup (165g) frozen corn
- 1 cup (160g) frozen peas

1. Preheat the oven to 370°F.
2. In a large pot over high heat, cover the potatoes in water and bring to a boil. Boil for 20 minutes, or until easily pierced with a fork.
3. Drain the potatoes and mash them, using a potato masher or fork, along with the coconut milk, coconut oil, 2 teaspoons of salt, and ¼ teaspoon of pepper, until completely combined and smooth.
4. Heat a large skillet over medium-high heat. Spray with cooking spray and add the ground turkey, breaking it apart with a wooden spoon. Add the oregano, parsley, basil, remaining ½ teaspoon of salt, and remaining ¼ teaspoon of pepper and continue to cook until evenly browned and no signs of pink are showing, about 10 minutes.
5. Coat an 11-by-14-inch baking dish with cooking spray. Spread the turkey over the bottom of the dish. Pour the mushroom soup over the top of the turkey, sprinkle the corn and peas on top, then spread evenly with the mashed potatoes.
6. Bake for 30 to 35 minutes, until lightly golden brown on top, then let cool.
7. Divide the shepherd's pie evenly among 8 airtight storage containers and seal.

PER SERVING

Calories: 467| Fat: 17g| Protein: 34g| Total Carbs: 47g| Net Carbs: 40g| Fiber: 7g| Sugar: 5g| Sodium: 863mg

Deconstructed Taco Bowls

Prep time: 5 minutes | Cook time: 15 minutes| Serves 4

- 2 (5-inch) hard corn taco shells (26g)
- 2 cups (500g) cooked rice
- Nonstick cooking spray
- ¾ pound (340g) extra-lean ground turkey
- 1 yellow onion (94g), chopped
- 2 tablespoons (35g) taco seasoning
- 1 cup (130g) salsa
- 1 cup (80g) canned black beans, rinsed and drained, divided
- 1 cup (80g) cooked corn kernels, divided
- ½ cup (249g) reduced-fat sour cream (5%), divided
- ¼ cup (4g) finely chopped fresh cilantro, divided
- 1 lime (67g), sliced into wedges, divided

1. Preheat the oven to 350°F.
2. Place the shells on a baking sheet and cook for 3 to 4 minutes.
3. Into each container, place ½ cup of cooked rice and set aside.
4. While the taco shells are in the oven, heat a large nonstick skillet over medium-high heat. Spray with cooking spray, and add the ground turkey and onion. Cook until browned, about 10 minutes. Remove from the heat, drain any liquid, place back on the heat, and stir in the taco seasoning.
5. Add the salsa and cook just until heated through and well combined. Remove from the heat.
6. In each container, top the rice with an equal amount of turkey, ¼ cup of black beans, ¼ cup of corn, 2 tablespoons of sour cream, and 1 tablespoon of cilantro. Garnish each with 2 slices of lime, and seal.
7. Place the taco shells in another container, seal, and store at room temperature until ready for use. When ready to serve, fill half a taco shell with the turkey rice mixture or simply crush it and sprinkle on top for a bit of extra crunch.

PER SERVING

Calories: 488| Fat: 13g| Protein: 27g| Total Carbs: 63g| Net Carbs: 57g| Fiber: 6g| Sugar: 10g| Sodium: 1151mg

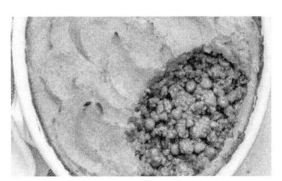

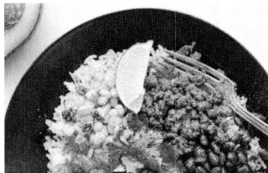

Green Beans Almondine

Prep time: 15 minutes | Cook time: 15 minutes| Serves 4

- Salt and ground black pepper, to taste
- 1 pound fresh green beans, trimmed
- 1/2 teaspoon extra-virgin olive oil
- 1/4 cup slivered almonds

1. Bring a large pot of lightly salted water to a boil over high heat. Add green beans and boil until tender, about 2 to 4 minutes.
2. Drain beans and transfer them to a large bowl. Drizzle with olive oil and season with salt and pepper; toss.
3. Warm a large nonstick skillet over medium-high heat. Coat almonds with cooking spray and add to the hot skillet. Stir frequently until toasted, about 2 to 3 minutes.
4. Reduce heat to medium and add the green beans. Cook for another 2 minutes, stirring occasionally. Remove from heat and serve.

PER SERVING

Calories:79 | protein: 3g| carbs: 10g|fat: 5g

Grilled Balsamic Vegetable Platter with Shaved Parmesan

Prep time: 25 minutes, plus 45 minutes to marinate | Cook time: 15 minutes| Serves 4

- 1/2 cup extra-virgin olive oil
- 2 tablespoons balsamic vinegar
- Salt and ground black pepper, to taste
- 2 eggplants, cut into 1/2-inch slices
- 3 zucchini, cut into 1/2-inch slices
- 2 yellow squash, cut into 1/2-inch slices
- 2 red bell peppers, seeded and cut into 1/2-inch slices
- 1/4 cup shaved Parmesan cheese

1. In a large bowl, whisk together olive oil, vinegar, salt, and pepper. Add eggplant, zucchini, squash, and bell peppers. Toss to coat and set aside for about 45 minutes to marinate.
2. Prepare a grill to medium heat. Lightly coat the grill grates with cooking spray. Using tongs, remove vegetables from marinade, shaking off the excess. Turning occasionally, grill vegetables until tender, 10 to 15 minutes, brushing them with the excess marinade every few minutes as they cook.
3. Transfer grilled vegetables to a platter. Garnish with Parmesan and serve.

PER SERVING

Calories:382 | protein: 8g| carbs: 26g|fat: 29g

Crispy Squash Fries

Prep time: 5 minutes | Cook time: 15 minutes| Serves 4

- 1 teaspoon extra-virgin olive oil
- 2 egg whites or 6 tablespoons liquid egg white substitute
- 1/2 cup skim milk
- 1/3 cup bread crumbs
- 1 tablespoon grated Parmesan cheese
- 1/2 teaspoon onion powder
- 1/2 teaspoon sweet paprika
- 1/2 teaspoon dried parsley
- 1/2 teaspoon garlic powder
- 1/4 teaspoon ground black pepper
- 2 large yellow squash, quartered lengthwise and then cut in half widthwise

1. Preheat the oven to 450 degrees F. Prepare a large baking dish by greasing with oil.
2. In a medium bowl, add egg whites and milk. Lightly whisk together.
3. In a separate medium bowl, combine breadcrumbs, cheese, onion powder, paprika, parsley, garlic powder, and pepper.
4. Place breaded squash cut-side-up into the prepared baking pan. Continue until all the squash has been breaded.
5. Bake squash in the oven until browned, about 15 minutes. Serve.

PER SERVING

Calories: 143| protein: 8g| carbs: 21g|fat: 3g

Sweet Potato Chips

Prep time: 5 minutes | Cook time: 25 minutes| Serves 6

- 2 medium sweet potatoes (5 ounces each), peeled and thinly sliced
- 1 tablespoon extra-virgin olive oil
- 1/2 teaspoon salt

1. Position one rack in the center of the oven and one in the lower position. Preheat the oven to 400 degrees F. Prepare 2 baking sheets by coating with cooking spray.
2. Add sweet potatoes to a large bowl and drizzle with olive oil. Toss to coat with tongs or clean hands. Spread potatoes in an even layer on both baking sheets and place in the oven.
3. Bake potatoes, flipping once halfway through cooking time, until centers are soft and edges are slightly crispy, about 22 to 25 minutes. Sprinkle with salt and serve.

PER SERVING

Calories: 61| protein: 1g| carbs: 10g|fat: 2g

Spiced Salmon with Roasted Broccoli and Cauliflower

Prep time: 5 minutes | Cook time: 40 minutes| Serves 6

- For the cauliflower and broccoli
- 1 broccoli head (318g), cut into florets
- 1 cauliflower head (575g), cut into florets
- Nonstick olive oil spray
- Sea salt
- Freshly ground black pepper
- Juice of ½ lemon (30ml)

FOR THE SALMON

- 1½ to 2 pounds (0.78 to 1.04kg) salmon fillet
- Nonstick olive oil spray
- ¼ teaspoon (0.7g) garlic powder
- ¼ teaspoon (0.6g) onion powder
- ½ teaspoon (1.1g) paprika
- ½ teaspoon (0.25g) dried parsley
- ½ teaspoon (0.35g) dried basil
- Pinch ground cayenne pepper
- Salt
- Freshly ground black pepper
- ½ lemon (42g), sliced

TO MAKE THE CAULIFLOWER AND BROCCOLI

1. Preheat the oven to 425°F.
2. In a large bowl, combine the broccoli and cauliflower. Spray liberally with olive oil, and season with salt and pepper.
3. Spread the vegetables out onto a sheet pan and bake for 20 minutes.
4. Remove from the oven, let cool, then toss with the lemon juice.
5. To make the salmon
6. Reduce the oven to 400°F.
7. Place the salmon on a roasting pan, skin-side down.
8. Spray liberally with olive oil, then season evenly with garlic powder, onion powder, paprika, parsley, basil, and cayenne pepper. Season with salt and pepper to taste, and top with the lemon slices.
9. Bake for 15 to 20 minutes, or until the fish flakes when pierced with a fork and is no longer translucent inside. Remove from the oven and let cool.
10. Divide the salmon and vegetables evenly among 6 airtight storage containers and seal.

PER SERVING

Calories: 379| Fat: 18g| Protein: 37g| Total Carbs: 10g| Net Carbs: 6g| Fiber: 4g| Sugar: 4g| Sodium: 156mg

Roasted Brussels Sprouts

Prep time: 15 minutes | Cook time: 45 minutes| Serves 4

- 1 1/2 pounds Brussels sprouts, ends trimmed and yellow leaves removed
- 3 tablespoons extra-virgin olive oil
- Salt and ground black pepper, to taste
- 1/4 cup chopped fresh cilantro

1. Preheat oven to 400 degrees F.
2. Place Brussels sprouts, olive oil, salt, and pepper into a large Ziploc bag. Seal tightly and shake to coat.
3. Pour onto a baking sheet and roast in the oven for 30 to 45 minutes. Shake the pan halfway through cooking for even browning. Brussels sprouts should be dark brown, almost black, when done.
4. Garnish with a sprinkling of chopped cilantro and serve immediately.

PER SERVING

Calories: 164| protein: 6g| carbs: 16g|fat: 11g

Brown Rice Pilaf

Prep time: 5 minutes | Cook time: 45 minutes, plus 10 minutes resting | Serves 4

- 1 tablespoon unsalted butter
- 1 shallot, peeled and finely chopped
- 1 cup long-grain brown rice, rinsed
- Salt and ground black pepper, to taste
- 2 cups low-sodium chicken broth
- 1 clove garlic, peeled and smashed
- 2 sprigs fresh thyme
- 3 tablespoons chopped fresh flat-leaf parsley
- 3 scallions, thinly sliced

1. Melt butter in a medium heavy-duty pot over medium heat. Add shallot and cook until tender, about 1 to 2 minutes.
2. Add rice, stirring well to coat with the butter and shallots. Cook for a few minutes until rice is glossy. Season with salt and pepper.
3. Stir in chicken broth, garlic, and thyme. Cover with a tight-fitting lid, reduce heat to low, and cook for 40 minutes. Remove from heat and let sit for 10 minutes.
4. Use a fork to fluff rice and stir in parsley and scallions. Serve.

PER SERVING

Calories: 218| protein: 5g| carbs: 39g|fat: 4g

Quinoa Salad with Almonds and Dried Cranberries

Prep time: 5 minutes , plus 10 minutes resting | Cook time: 20 minutes| Serves 4

- 1 1/2 cups water
- 1 cup dry quinoa, rinsed
- 1/2 cup grated carrots
- 1/4 cup chopped red bell pepper
- 1/4 cup chopped yellow bell pepper
- 1 small red onion, finely chopped
- 1 1/2 teaspoons curry powder
- 1/4 cup chopped fresh cilantro
- Juice of 1 lime
- 1/4 cup almonds slivers, toasted
- 1/2 cup dried cranberries
- Salt and ground black pepper, to taste

1. Add water into a medium, heavy-duty pot, cover with a tight-fitting lid, and warm over high heat. Once water boils, stir in quinoa. Reduce heat to low, and cover.
2. Simmer until quinoa absorbs the water, about 15 to 20 minutes. Transfer quinoa to a large bowl and refrigerate until cool.
3. Once quinoa has chilled, stir in carrots, bell peppers, onion, curry, cilantro, lime juice, almonds, cranberries, salt, and pepper. Toss and serve.

PER SERVING

Calories:310 | protein: 9g| carbs: 56g|fat: 6g

Garlicky Zucchini and Spinach Sauté

Prep time: 5 minutes | Cook time: 15 minutes| Serves 6

- 1 tablespoon extra-virgin olive oil
- 2 cloves garlic, peeled and minced
- 2 zucchini, cut into matchsticks
- 2 cups grape tomatoes
- 3 cups baby spinach
- 1 tablespoon lemon juice
- Pinch of ground black pepper

1. Warm oil in a large pan over medium-low heat. Add garlic and cook until fragrant, about 1 minute. Add zucchini and increase the heat to medium. Cook for 3 to 4 minutes, stirring constantly.
2. Stir in tomatoes, cooking for 1 minute. Add spinach, stirring and sautéing for another 3 to 4 minutes until wilted. Add lemon juice and black pepper before removing from heat to serve.

PER SERVING

Calories: 46| protein: 2g| carbs: 5g|fat: 2g

Roasted Garlic Twice-Baked Potato

Prep time: 25 minutes | Cook time: 1 hour 25 minutes| Serves 6

- 6 medium baking potatoes (8 ounces each), poked with a few holes
- 1 whole garlic bulb
- 1 teaspoon extra-virgin olive oil
- 2 tablespoons unsalted butter, softened
- 1/2 cup skim milk
- 1/2 cup buttermilk
- 1 1/2 teaspoons finely chopped fresh rosemary leaves
- 1/2 teaspoon salt
- 1/2 teaspoon ground black pepper
- Sweet paprika, to taste

1. Preheat oven to 400 degrees F. Place potatoes onto a baking sheet and cook in the oven until fork-tender, about 1 hour.
2. Meanwhile, remove the outer papery skin from garlic bulb, drizzle with oil, and wrap in 2 sheets of heavy-duty foil. Bake the garlic in the 400 degrees F oven until softened, about 30 to 35 minutes. Allow garlic and potatoes to cool for about 10 minutes.
3. Increase the oven's temperature to 425 degrees F.
4. Once cool enough to handle, cut a thin slice off the top of each potato and discard. Scoop out potato flesh until a thin shell remains. Add potato flesh into a large bowl along with butter; mash together.
5. Cut the top off the garlic bulb, leaving the root intact, and squeeze roasted garlic into the potato mixture. Add milk, buttermilk, rosemary, salt, and pepper. Mix well.
6. Spoon the potato mixture back into the potato skins and return to the baking sheet. Bake until heated through, about 20 to 25 minutes. Remove from oven and garnish with a dash of paprika.

PER SERVING

Calories:242 | protein: 6g| carbs: 43g|fat: 6g

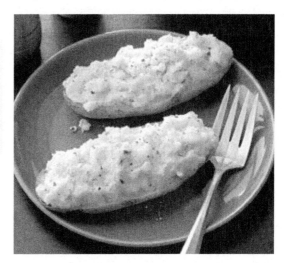

Curried Potatoes and Cauliflower

Prep time: 5 minutes | Cook time: 25 minutes| Serves 4

- Salt, to taste
- 1 (2- to 3-pound) head cauliflower, cut into florets
- 1 pound potatoes, peeled and cut into 1-inch cubes
- 1 medium onion, chopped
- 2 cloves garlic, peeled and minced
- 2 tablespoons garam masala or curry powder
- 1 cup low-sodium vegetable broth
- 2 cups frozen peas

1. Bring a pot of lightly salted water to a boil over high heat. Add the cauliflower and potatoes; cook for 4 to 5 minutes and drain.
2. Meanwhile, coat a Dutch oven with cooking spray and warm over medium heat. Add chopped onion and garlic and cook until onion softens, about 2 to 3 minutes. Add garam masala and stir for 1 minute.
3. Transfer cooked potatoes and cauliflower to the Dutch oven. Stir well, coating in the onion mixture. Add broth and deglaze the pan.
4. Cover with a lid and let mixture simmer for 10 minutes. Stir in peas, cover, and cook for another 5 to 7 minutes. Serve immediately.

PER SERVING

Calories:230 | protein: 12g| carbs: 47g|fat: 1g

Butternut Squash and Broccoli Stir-Fry

Prep time: 15 minutes | Cook time: 15 minutes| Serves 6

- 1 pound butternut squash, peeled, seeded, and cut into 1/4-inch slices
- 1 clove garlic, peeled and minced
- 1/4 teaspoon ground ginger
- 1 cup broccoli florets
- 1/2 cup thinly sliced celery
- 1/2 cup thinly sliced onion
- 2 teaspoons honey
- 1 tablespoon lemon juice
- 2 tablespoons sunflower seed kernels

1. Coat a large skillet with cooking spray and warm over medium-high heat. Add squash, garlic, and ginger; stir-fry for 3 minutes.
2. Add broccoli, celery, and onion and continue to stir-fry until vegetables are tender, about 3 to 4 minutes.
3. Meanwhile, in a small bowl, combine honey and lemon juice. Mix well.
4. Transfer vegetables to a large serving dish and pour the honey mixture over top. Using tongs, toss to coat. Garnish with sunflower kernels and serve.

PER SERVING

Calories:71 | protein: 2g| carbs: 14g|fat: 2g

Lean Rice Crispy Treats

Prep time 25 minutes | Cook time 5 minutes| Serves 12

- ⅔ cup natural almond butter
- ½ cup raw honey
- ½ cup vanilla whey protein powder
- 1 tbsp ground cinnamon
- 3 cups toasted brown rice cereal

1. In a large glass bowl, combine the almond butter and honey. Warm in the microwave on medium for 30 to 45 seconds, stir, then add the protein powder and cinnamon. Stir well.
2. Add the brown rice cereal and gently fold it into the mixture. Pour into a 9 x 13in (23 x 33cm) baking dish and use a spoon to flatten the mixture and form a uniform surface.
3. Place in the refrigerator to harden for 15 minutes before cutting into 12 equal-sized squares.

PER SERVING

Calories:183 |fat:8.4g|carbs: 20g| protein: 8.6g

Bison and Portobello Sliders

Prep time 30 minutes | Cook time 15 minutes| Serves 2

- 1lb (450g) lean ground bison, preferably 92/8 lean-
- ¼ cup liquid egg whites
- 2 tbsp dried onion flakes
- 1 tsp garlic powder
- ½ tsp salt
- ½ tsp ground black pepper
- 4 tbsp no-sugar-added ketchup (optional)
- 8 large portobello mushrooms
- ½ tsp salt
- ½ tsp ground black pepper
- ½ tsp garlic powder

1. Preheat the grill to medium. In a large bowl, combine the ground bison, egg whites, onion flakes, garlic powder, salt, and black pepper. Mix until the ingredients are well incorporated. With wet hands, shape the mixture into 8 even-sized patties. Set aside.
2. Rinse the mushrooms and pat dry with a paper towel. Remove the stems and place on a flat surface, gill-sides up. Season with the salt, black pepper, and garlic powder.
3. Place the mushrooms on the grill, gill-sides up, and grill for 3 minutes. Flip and grill for an additional 2 to 3 minutes. Transfer to a paper towel to drain, gill-sides down.
4. Place the bison patties on the grill, and cook for 4 to 5 minutes per side. Transfer to a plate and allow to rest for 5 minutes. Assemble the sliders by placing a bison patty between two portobello buns. Top each slider with 1 tbsp ketchup (if using). Serve warm.

PER SERVING

Calories:212 |fat:9g|carbs: 9g| protein: 27g

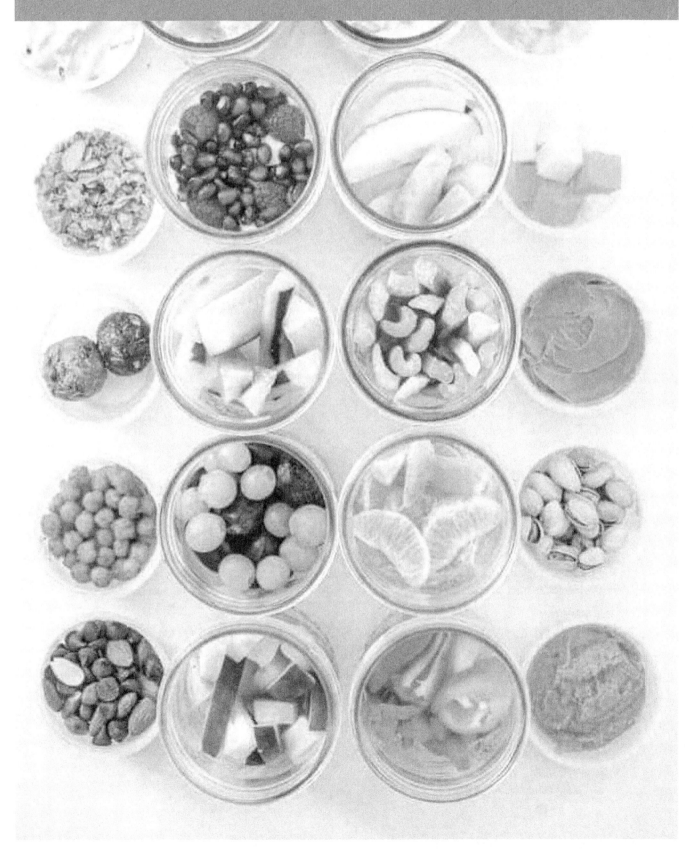

Chapter 13
Sweets and Snacks

Dark Chocolate Peanut Butter Cups

Prep time: 10 minutes| **Cook time:** 1 to 2 minutes, plus 15 minutes to chill| **Makes 12 peanut butter cups**

- 1 cup (182 grams) dark chocolate chips
- 1 cup (98 grams) peanut butter powder
- ¾ cup (177 milliliters) water

1. Line a 12-cup muffin tin with ridged, silicone liners.
2. In a microwave-safe bowl, heat the chocolate chips in 30-second intervals until melted, stirring between each interval.
3. Spoon about 2 teaspoons of chocolate into each cup.
4. In a small bowl, mix the peanut butter powder and water until smooth. Divide the mixture between the cups, about 1 tablespoon in each.
5. Reheat the remaining chocolate in the microwave until smooth and melted. Top each cup with the remaining melted chocolate, about 2 teaspoons each.
6. Place the cups in the refrigerator for about 15 minutes to set.

PER SERVING (1 PEANUT BUTTER CUP)

Calories: 121| Fat: 7g| Protein: 4g| Total Carbs: 11g| Fiber: 3g| Sugar: 7g| Sodium: 48mg

Broiled Grapefruit with Greek Yogurt and Pecans

Prep time: 5 minutes | **Cook time:** 15 minutes| **Serves 2**

- 2 grapefruit (512 grams), halved
- 4 packed tablespoons (55 grams) brown sugar
- 2 cups (490 grams) nonfat plain Greek yogurt
- ¼ cup (27 grams) pecan pieces
- 2 tablespoons (42 grams) honey

1. Preheat the broiler on high.
2. Place the grapefruit, cut-side up, on a baking sheet and sprinkle each half with 1 tablespoon of brown sugar.
3. Broil for about 10 minutes, until the sugar caramelizes and is bubbling. Top each half with ½ cup of yogurt, 1 tablespoon of pecan pieces, and ½ tablespoon of honey. Serve warm.

PER SERVING

Calories: 515| Fat: 11g| Protein: 28g| Total Carbs: 82g| Fiber: 5g| Sugar: 70g| Sodium: 97mg

Almond Butter Protein Bites

Prep time: 5 minutes | **Cook time:** 5 minutes| **Makes 24 bites**

- ½ cup (88 grams) pitted dates
- ½ cup (118 milliliters) maple syrup
- ¼ cup (60 grams) almond butter
- ¼ cup (30 grams) ground flaxseed
- 2 scoops (68 grams) whey protein powder
- 1 cup (80 grams) rolled oats
- 2 tablespoons (23 grams) dark chocolate chips

1. In a food processor, combine the dates, maple syrup, almond butter, flaxseed, and whey and pulse to combine and break up the dates.
2. Add the oats and pulse until the dates are finely chopped. Stir in the chocolate chips.
3. Using your hands, shape the mixture into 24 balls, about 1 inch in diameter.

PER SERVING (2 BITES)

Calories: 160| Fat: 5g| Protein: 7g| Total Carbs: 22g| Fiber: 3g| Sugar: 14g| Sodium: 19mg

High-Protein Crab Balls

Prep time: 15 minutes | **Cook time:** 20 minutes| **Serves 4**

- Nonstick cooking spray
- 1 pound (453 grams) crab meat
- 1 cup (80 grams) panko bread crumbs
- 1 large egg (50 grams), beaten
- 2 tablespoons (30 milliliters) lemon juice
- 1 scallion (15 grams), sliced, both white and green parts
- ½ teaspoon (1.2 grams) Old Bay seasoning
- ¼ teaspoon (0.58 gram) freshly ground black pepper

1. Preheat the oven to 375°F. Line a baking sheet with parchment paper and coat with cooking spray.
2. In a small bowl, mix the crab, bread crumbs, egg, lemon juice, scallion, Old Bay seasoning, and pepper and mix well. Form the mixture into 12 balls, place them on the prepared baking sheet, and coat lightly with cooking spray.
3. Bake for 20 minutes, until lightly browned. Serve warm or chilled.

PER SERVING

Calories: 184| Fat: 2g| Protein: 24g| Total Carbs: 17g| Fiber: 1g| Sugar: 2g| Sodium: 632mg

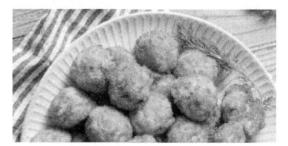

Peanut Butter Oat Protein Bars

Prep time: 15 minutes | Cook time: 20 minutes|Makes 8 bars

- ½ cup (128 grams) creamy peanut butter
- ½ cup (118 milliliters) non-dairy milk
- ½ cup (118 milliliters) maple syrup
- 2 cups (162 grams) rolled oats
- ¼ cup (28 grams) ground flaxseed
- ¼ cup (26 grams) peanut butter powder
- ½ teaspoon (1.32 grams) ground cinnamon

1. Line an 8-inch baking dish with parchment paper.
2. In a medium pot over medium heat, heat the peanut butter, milk, and maple syrup until peanut butter is melted and milk is steaming.
3. Add the oats, flaxseed, peanut butter powder, and cinnamon and mix until well combined.
4. Press the mixture into the prepared baking dish in an even layer. Let cool to room temperature, then cut into 8 pieces.
5. Store in an airtight container in the refrigerator for up to one week.

PER SERVING (1 BAR)

Calories: 261| Fat: 11g| Protein: 9g| Total Carbs: 34g| Fiber: 4g| Sugar: 14g| Sodium: 104mg

Stuffed Avocado

Prep time: 10 minutes | Cook time: 5 minutes| Serves 2

- 1 (15-ounce) can (425 grams) black beans, drained and rinsed
- 1 (15-ounce) can (425 grams) sweet corn, drained
- 1 Roma tomato (53 grams), diced
- 2 tablespoons (2 grams) chopped cilantro
- Juice of 1 lime (29 milliliters)
- 1 garlic clove (3 grams), minced
- Pinch salt
- Freshly ground black pepper
- 1 small avocado (150 grams), halved and pitted

1. In a small bowl, mix the black beans, corn, tomato, and cilantro. Add the lime juice and garlic, then season with salt and pepper.
2. Divide the bean salad between the avocado halves and serve.

PER SERVING

Calories: 449| Fat: 14g| Protein: 18g| Total Carbs: 71g| Fiber: 25g| Sugar: 8g| Sodium: 303mg

Coconut-Cranberry Trail Mix

Prep time: 5 minutes | Cook time: 5 minutes| Serves 4

- 6 ounces (170 grams) whole-grain pretzels
- 1 cup (160 grams) dried cranberries
- ½ cup (40 grams) coconut flakes
- ¼ cup (34 grams) shelled sunflower seeds
- ¼ cup (30 grams) raw almonds
- ¼ cup (29 grams) walnut pieces

1. In a bowl, combine the pretzels, cranberries, coconut, sunflower seeds, almonds, and walnuts.
2. Mix well and store in an airtight container at room temperature for up to one month.

PER SERVING

Calories: 323| Fat: 14g| Protein: 7g| Total Carbs: 50g| Fiber: 7g| Sugar: 20g| Sodium: 62mg

Blueberry Peanut Butter Muffins

Prep time: 5 minutes | Cook time: 20 minutes| Makes 12 muffins

- Nonstick cooking spray
- 1 cup (245 grams) nonfat plain Greek yogurt
- ½ cup (125 grams) unsweetened apple sauce
- ⅓ cup (79 milliliters) maple syrup
- ¼ cup (59 milliliters) skim milk
- 2 tablespoons (30 milliliters) avocado oil
- 2 large eggs (100 grams)
- 2 cups (240 grams) oat flour
- ¼ cup (26 grams) peanut butter powder
- 1 teaspoon (4 grams) baking powder
- 1 cup (148 grams) fresh or frozen blueberries

1. Preheat the oven to 350°F. Line a 12-cup muffin tin with ridged, silicone liners.
2. In a large bowl, combine the yogurt, applesauce, maple syrup, milk, oil, and eggs.
3. Add the oat flour, peanut butter powder, and baking powder, and mix well.
4. Fold in the blueberries.
5. Spoon the batter evenly into the muffin tin. Bake for 20 minutes, until a toothpick inserted in the center comes out clean.

PER SERVING (1 MUFFIN)

Calories: 167| Fat: 5g| Protein: 7g| Total Carbs: 24g| Fiber: 3g| Sugar: 9g| Sodium: 78mg

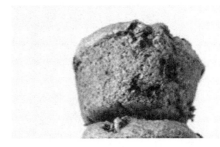

Homemade Granola

Prep time: 5 minutes | Cook time: 25 minutes| Serves 8

- 3 cups (243 grams) rolled oats
- 1 cup (118 grams) pepitas
- ½ teaspoon (1.32 grams) ground cinnamon
- ½ cup (125 grams) unsweetened apple sauce
- ¼ cup (60 milliliters) maple syrup
- 2 teaspoons (10 milliliters) vanilla extract

1. Preheat the oven to 300°F. Line a large baking sheet with parchment paper.
2. In a large bowl, combine the oats, pepitas, and cinnamon and mix well. Stir in the applesauce, maple syrup, and vanilla and mix well.
3. Spread the mixture on the baking sheet in an even layer. Bake for 25 minutes, stirring every 5 minutes, until toasted and browned.
4. Let cool on the baking tray| then break apart to store in an airtight container for up to two weeks.

PER SERVING

Calories: 233| Fat: 9g| Protein: 8g| Total Carbs: 31g| Fiber: 4g| Sugar: 8g| Sodium: 6mg

Garlicky Chili-Chive Popcorn

Prep time: 10 minutes | Cook time: 2 minutes | Serves 4

- 2½ tablespoons olive oil, divided
- ½ cup popcorn kernels
- ½ teaspoon garlic powder
- ½ teaspoon onion powder
- 3 tablespoons minced fresh chives
- 2 tablespoons nutritional yeast
- ¼ teaspoon sea salt
- ¼ teaspoon chili flakes (optional)

1. Heat 2 tablespoons of olive oil in a large pot over medium heat. Add the popcorn kernels, cover, and cook, shaking the pot often, until there are 3 seconds between pops and most of the kernels have popped. Transfer the popcorn to a large bowl.
2. Heat the remaining ½ tablespoon of olive oil in a very small saucepan over medium heat. Add the garlic powder and onion powder and cook, stirring constantly, for about 1 minute.
3. Pour the seasoned oil over the popcorn and mix well. Add the chives, nutritional yeast, salt, and chili flakes, if using, and toss until evenly coated.
4. Divide the popcorn equally into 4 bowls.

PER SERVING

Calories: 203 | Fat: 10 g | Protein: 6 g | Sodium: 386 mg | Fiber: 5 g | Carbohydrates: 24 g | Sugar: 8g

Bagel Seasoning with Roasted Edamame

Prep time: 10 minutes | Cook time: 40 minutes | Serves 4

- 1 teaspoon white sesame seeds
- ½ teaspoon black sesame seeds
- ½ teaspoon dried garlic
- ½ teaspoon dried onion
- ½ teaspoon sea salt
- ¼ teaspoon poppy seeds
- 2 teaspoons olive oil

1. Preheat the oven to 375°F (190°C). Line a baking sheet with parchment paper.
2. Put the frozen edamame in a colander and quickly run them under warm water to remove any ice. Pat the edamame dry using a clean dish towel and set aside for 20 minutes to dry completely.
3. While the edamame is drying, in a small bowl, mix the white and black sesame seeds, garlic, onion, salt, and poppy seeds.
4. In a large mixing bowl, toss together the dried edamame and olive oil until evenly coated. Add the seasoning mixture and mix well. Spread out the seasoned edamame on the prepared baking sheet. Avoid overcrowding.
5. Roast for 35 to 40 minutes, stirring every 10 minutes, or until crispy. Transfer the edamame to a bowl and serve. Refrigerate any leftovers in an airtight container for up to 3 days.

PER SERVING

Calories: 158 | Fat: 8 g | Protein: 12 g | Sodium: 240 mg | Fiber: 6 g | Carbohydrates: 11 g | Sugar: 3 g

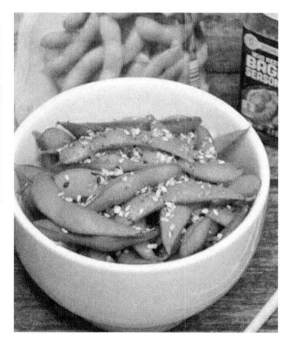

Garlic Turmeric Roasted Chickpeas

Prep time: 5 minutes | Cook time: 35 minutes | Serves 4

- 1 (15-ounce (425g) can chickpeas, drained and rinsed
- ½ teaspoon ground turmeric
- ½ teaspoon garlic powder
- ½ teaspoon sea salt
- ¼ teaspoon freshly ground black pepper
- 2 teaspoons olive oil

1. Preheat the oven to 375°F (190°C). Line a baking sheet with parchment paper.
2. Pat the chickpeas dry with a clean kitchen towel. Spread out the dried chickpeas on the prepared baking sheet. Avoid overcrowding. Let the chickpeas dry for at least 15 minutes.
3. Bake for 30 to 35 minutes, shaking the baking sheet every 10 minutes, or until the chickpeas are a light golden brown.
4. While the chickpeas are baking, in a small bowl, mix the turmeric, garlic powder, salt, and pepper.
5. Transfer the roasted chickpeas to a medium bowl. Add the olive oil and toss until evenly coated. Add the seasoning and toss until evenly coated.
6. Store any leftovers in a container for up to 4 days. Cover loosely to maintain crispiness.

PER SERVING

Calories: 101 | Fat: 4 g | Protein: 4 g | Sodium: 354 mg | Fiber: 4 g | Carbohydrates: 14 g | Sugar: 5g

Lemon and Almond Snack Mix

Prep time: 10 minutes | Cook time: 3 minutes | Serves 4

- 1 tablespoon reduced-sodium soy sauce
- 1 tablespoon freshly squeezed lemon juice
- ⅛ teaspoon onion powder
- ⅛ teaspoon garlic powder
- ⅛ teaspoon cayenne pepper
- ¼ cup raw pepitas
- ⅓ cup whole almonds
- ⅓ cup unsalted cashews
- ½ cup unsalted air-popped popcorn
- ½ cup unsalted mini pretzel sticks

1. In a small bowl, mix the soy sauce, lemon juice, onion powder, garlic powder, and cayenne pepper. Set aside.
2. In a large skillet over medium-low heat, combine the pepitas, almonds, and cashews and cook, stirring frequently, until toasted, 2 to 3 minutes. Immediately drizzle with the soy sauce mixture and remove the pan from the heat. Add the popcorn and pretzels and stir until evenly coated. Transfer the mixture to a large bowl and serve immediately.
3. Store any leftover snack mix in an airtight container for up to 3 days.

PER SERVING

Calories: 233 | Fat: 15 g | Protein: 8 g | Sodium: 167 mg | Fiber: 0 g | Carbohydrates: 19 g | Sugar: 7g

Nutritional Peppered Kale Chips

Prep time: 5 minutes | Cook time: 18 minutes | Serves 4

- 6 ounces (170g) kale, stemmed, washed, and dried
- 2 teaspoons olive oil
- 1½ tablespoons nutritional yeast
- ¼ teaspoon sea salt
- ½ teaspoon freshly ground black pepper

1. Preheat the oven to 225°F (107°C). Line a baking sheet with parchment paper.
2. In a large bowl, mix the kale and olive oil until evenly coated. Put the kale onto the prepared baking sheet.
3. Sprinkle the nutritional yeast, salt, and pepper over the kale.
4. Bake for 15 minutes, or until the edges of the kale are slightly brown. To increase the crispiness, rotate the pan and continue to bake for another 3 to 5 minutes. Watch closely to avoid burning.
5. Let the kale chips cool on the pan for 2 minutes to increase the crispiness. Transfer to a large bowl and let cool completely before serving.

PER SERVING

Calories: 53 | Fat: 3 g | Protein: 3 g | Sodium: 332 mg | Fiber: 2 g | Carbohydrates: 5 g | Sugar: 4 g

Baked Chewy Banana Bites

Prep time: 10 minutes | Cook time: 15 minutes | Serves 12

- ¼ cup whole unsalted almonds
- 2 large ripe bananas
- 1 cup plus 2 tablespoons rolled oats
- 4 teaspoons hemp hearts
- 2 tablespoons ground flaxseed
- 1 tablespoon vanilla extract
- 2 teaspoons ground cinnamon
- ⅛ teaspoon sea salt
- 2½ tablespoons 70% dark chocolate chips

1. Preheat the oven to 350°F (180°C). Line a baking sheet with parchment paper.
2. Put the almonds in a small zip-top plastic bag, seal, and crush them using a rolling pin.
3. In a large bowl, mash the bananas with a fork. Add the oats, hemp hearts, flaxseed, almonds, vanilla, cinnamon, and salt and mix well. Add the chocolate chips and mix until well combined.
4. Using your hands, form the mixture into 12 equal balls and place them on the prepared baking sheet. Using a spoon, gently press down on each ball to flatten the tops.
5. Bake for 15 minutes, or until slightly golden. Let the bites cool on a wire rack for 10 minutes before serving.
6. Store any leftover bites in an airtight container for up to 3 days.

PER SERVING

Calories: 95 | Fat: 4 g | Protein: 3 g | Sodium: 21 mg | Fiber: 3 g | Carbohydrates: 13g | Sugar:9 g

Vanilla Chocolate Graham Cracker Cups

Prep time: 10 minutes | Cook time: 1 minute | Serves 6

- ½ cup pitted dates
- 1 teaspoon vanilla extract
- ¼ cup crushed graham crackers plus 1 tablespoon for sprinkling
- 2 tablespoons ground flaxseed
- 1 teaspoon maple syrup
- 1 cup nonfat plain Greek yogurt
- 1 tablespoon 70% dark chocolate chips

1. Line a 6-cup muffin tin with liners. Set aside.
2. In a small bowl, soak the dates in hot water for 10 minutes. Drain well.
3. In a food processor, combine the soaked dates and vanilla and pulse until it forms a jamlike consistency. You may need to stop and scrape down the sides with a rubber spatula a few times. Transfer the mixture to a large bowl.
4. Add ¼ cup of graham crumbles, ground flaxseed, and maple syrup and stir until combined. Divide the mixture equally among the muffin cups and press it down to form a crust. Divide the Greek yogurt equally over the crust.
5. In a microwave-safe bowl, microwave the chocolate chips for 25 seconds, stir, and microwave again for 25 seconds. Continue to do this until the chocolate is melted and smooth.
6. Using a spoon, quickly drizzle the chocolate over the muffin cups. Sprinkle the remaining 1 tablespoon graham crumble over the cups. Freeze the pan for at least 30 minutes.
7. When ready to eat, let the graham cracker cups sit at room temperature for 5 minutes before serving.
8. Freeze any leftover cups in an airtight container, using parchment paper to separate them if needed, for up to 2 weeks.

PER SERVING

Calories: 147 | Fat: 3 g | Protein: 8 g | Sodium: 49 mg | Fiber: 3 g | Carbohydrates: 23 g | Sugar: 7 g

Chili-Chive Popcorn

Prep time: 5 minutes | Cook time: 10 minutes | Serves 4

- 2½ tablespoons olive oil, divided
- ½ cup popcorn kernels
- ½ teaspoon garlic powder
- ½ teaspoon onion powder
- 3 tablespoons minced fresh chives
- 2 tablespoons nutritional yeast
- ¼ teaspoon sea salt
- ¼ teaspoon chili flakes (optional)

1. Heat 2 tablespoons of olive oil in a large pot over medium heat. Add the popcorn kernels, cover, and cook, shaking the pot often, until there are 3 seconds between pops and most of the kernels have popped. Transfer the popcorn to a large bowl.

2. Heat the remaining ½ tablespoon of olive oil in a very small saucepan over medium heat. Add the garlic powder and onion powder and cook, stirring constantly, for about 1 minute.
3. Pour the seasoned oil over the popcorn and mix well. Add the chives, nutritional yeast, salt, and chili flakes, if using, and toss until evenly coated.
4. Divide the popcorn equally into 4 bowls.

PER SERVING

Calories: 203| Fat: 10g| Total Carbohydrates: 24g| Net Carbs: 19g| Fiber: 5g| Protein: 6g| Sodium: 386mg

Cheesy Peppered Kale Chips

Prep time: 5 minutes | Cook time: 20 minutes | Serves 4

- 6 ounces kale, stemmed, washed, and dried
- 2 teaspoons olive oil
- 1½ tablespoons nutritional yeast
- ¼ teaspoon sea salt
- ½ teaspoon freshly ground black pepper

1. Preheat the oven to 225°F. Line a baking sheet with parchment paper.
2. In a large bowl, mix the kale and olive oil until evenly coated. Put the kale onto the prepared baking sheet.
3. Sprinkle the nutritional yeast, salt, and pepper over the kale.
4. Bake for 15 minutes, or until the edges of the kale are slightly brown. To increase the crispiness, rotate the pan and continue to bake for another 3 to 5 minutes. Watch closely to avoid burning.
5. Let the kale chips cool on the pan for 2 minutes to increase the crispiness. Transfer to a large bowl and let cool completely before serving.

PER SERVING

Calories: 53| Fat: 3g| Total Carbohydrates: 5g| Net Carbs: 3g| Fiber: 2g| Protein: 3g| Sodium: 332mg

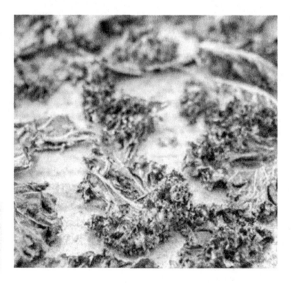

Roasted Edamame with Everything Bagel Seasoning

Prep time: 5 minutes, plus 20 minutes drying time | Cook time: 35 minutes| Serves 4

- 15 ounces frozen shelled edamame, rinsed and dried
- 1 teaspoon white sesame seeds
- ½ teaspoon black sesame seeds
- ½ teaspoon dried garlic
- ½ teaspoon dried onion
- ½ teaspoon sea salt
- ¼ teaspoon poppy seeds
- 2 teaspoons olive oil

1. Preheat the oven to 375°F. Line a baking sheet with parchment paper.
2. Put the frozen edamame in a colander and quickly run them under warm water to remove any ice. Pat the edamame dry using a clean dish towel and set aside for 20 minutes to dry completely.
3. While the edamame is drying, in a small bowl, mix the white and black sesame seeds, garlic, onion, salt, and poppy seeds.
4. In a large mixing bowl, toss together the dried edamame and olive oil until evenly coated. Add the seasoning mixture and mix well. Spread out the seasoned edamame on the prepared baking sheet. Avoid overcrowding.
5. Roast for 35 to 40 minutes, stirring every 10 minutes, or until crispy. Transfer the edamame to a bowl and serve. Refrigerate any leftovers in an airtight container for up to 3 days.

PER SERVING

Calories: 158| Fat: 8g| Total Carbohydrates: 11g| Net Carbs: 5g| Fiber: 6g| Protein: 12g| Sodium: 240mg

Peanut Butter Protein Swirl Brownies

Prep time: 15 minutes | Cook time: 25 minutes| Serves 10

BATTER

- 1 (15-ounce) can garbanzo beans, drained and rinsed
- 2 large eggs
- 2 tablespoons unsweetened cocoa powder
- 1/4 cup coconut sugar
- 1/2 teaspoon salt
- 2 tablespoons peanut butter
- 2 teaspoons vanilla extract
- 1 scoop unflavored whey protein
- 6 ounces dark chocolate, chopped, or 1 cup dark chocolate chips

TOPPING

- 1/2 cup 2% Greek yogurt
- 2 tablespoons egg whites or liquid egg white substitute
- 1 teaspoon vanilla extract
- 2 tablespoons peanut butter
- 1 scoop unflavored whey protein
- 1 teaspoon honey

1. Preheat the oven to 350 degrees F. Prepare an 8-inch by 8-inch baking pan by coating with cooking spray.
2. Into a blender or food processor, add garbanzo beans, eggs, cocoa powder, coconut sugar, salt, peanut butter, vanilla, and whey protein. Blend the ingredients until smooth. Transfer brownie batter to a medium bowl.
3. Using either a microwave or double boiler on the stove, gently stir the chocolate until melted. Stirring constantly, slowly pour the melted chocolate into the brownie batter. Use a spatula to evenly spread into the prepared pan. Set aside.
4. In a small bowl, add the topping ingredients and mix to combine. Pour topping over the brownie batter. Gently drag the tip of a knife through the mixture to create brownie swirls.
5. Bake brownies until topping is set and edges are golden brown, about 20 to 25 minutes. Let cool slightly and cut into 10 pieces. Store in an airtight container.

PER SERVING

Calories: 234| protein: 12g| carbs: 25g|fat: 11g

Turmeric Roasted Chickpeas

Prep time: 5 minutes, plus 15 minutes drying time | Cook time: 35 minutes| Serves 4

- 1 (15-ounce) can chickpeas, drained and rinsed
- ½ teaspoon ground turmeric
- ½ teaspoon garlic powder
- ½ teaspoon sea salt
- ¼ teaspoon freshly ground black pepper
- 2 teaspoons olive oil

1. Preheat the oven to 375°F. Line a baking sheet with parchment paper.
2. Pat the chickpeas dry with a clean kitchen towel. Spread out the dried chickpeas on the prepared baking sheet. Avoid overcrowding. Let the chickpeas dry for at least 15 minutes.
3. Bake for 30 to 35 minutes, shaking the baking sheet every 10 minutes, or until the chickpeas are a light golden brown.
4. While the chickpeas are baking, in a small bowl, mix the turmeric, garlic powder, salt, and pepper.
5. Transfer the roasted chickpeas to a medium bowl. Add the olive oil and toss until evenly coated. Add the seasoning and toss until evenly coated.
6. Store any leftovers in a container for up to 4 days. Cover loosely to maintain crispiness.

PER SERVING

Calories: 101| Fat: 4g| Total Carbohydrates: 14g| Net Carbs: 10g| Fiber: 4g| Protein: 4g| Sodium: 354mg

Spicy Snack Mix

Prep time: 5 minutes | Cook time: 5 minutes | Serves 4

- 1 tablespoon reduced-sodium soy sauce
- 1 tablespoon freshly squeezed lemon juice
- ⅛ teaspoon onion powder
- ⅛ teaspoon garlic powder
- ⅛ teaspoon cayenne pepper
- ¼ cup raw pepitas
- ⅓ cup whole almonds
- ⅓ cup unsalted cashews
- ½ cup unsalted air-popped popcorn
- ½ cup unsalted mini pretzel sticks

1. In a small bowl, mix the soy sauce, lemon juice, onion powder, garlic powder, and cayenne pepper. Set aside.
2. In a large skillet over medium-low heat, combine the pepitas, almonds, and cashews and cook, stirring frequently, until toasted, 2 to 3 minutes. Immediately drizzle with the soy sauce mixture and remove the pan from the heat. Add the popcorn and pretzels and stir until evenly coated. Transfer the mixture to a large bowl and serve immediately.
3. Store any leftover snack mix in an airtight container for up to 3 days.

PER SERVING

Calories: 233| Fat: 15g| Total Carbohydrates: 19g| Net Carbs: 16g| Fiber: 3g| Protein: 8g| Sodium: 167mg

Iced Pumpkin-Pecan Protein Bars

Prep time: 20 minutes | Cook time: 25 minutes, plus time to cool | Serves 9

BARS

- 4 large eggs
- 1 cup pumpkin purée
- 1/4 cup pure maple syrup
- 2 tablespoons unsweetened almond milk
- 1 teaspoon vanilla extract
- 1/3 cup coconut flour
- 2 scoops vanilla whey protein powder
- 2 tablespoons ground flaxseed
- 2 teaspoons ground cinnamon
- 1/4 teaspoon baking soda
- 1/2 teaspoon ground nutmeg
- 1/4 teaspoon sea salt
- 1/8 teaspoon ground cloves

TOPPING

- 1 scoop vanilla protein powder
- Room temperature water, as needed
- 1/4 cup chopped pecans

1. Preheat the oven to 375 degrees F. Prepare a baking sheet by lining with parchment paper or a silicone mat.
2. In a large bowl, add eggs, pumpkin, maple syrup,

almond milk, and vanilla. Use a fork to whisk together until combined.
3. In a medium bowl, add coconut flour, protein powder, flaxseed, cinnamon, baking soda, nutmeg, salt, and cloves, stirring together to combine.
4. Slowly stir dry ingredients into the pumpkin mixture until well combined; let sit for 2 to 3 minutes.
5. Separate batter into 8 parts, about 1/3 cup each. Form batter into rectangular bars by hand (like Clif bars) and place onto the prepared baking sheet.
6. Bake bars until golden brown on the bottom with a top just beginning to crack, about 22 to 25 minutes. Let bars cool for 5 minutes and then transfer to a wire rack.
7. Once bars have fully cooled, prepare the icing. Add protein powder to a small bowl, slowly stirring in water until mixture is thick and smooth.
8. Transfer icing into a small Ziploc bag and use scissors to cut off a small piece of the corner. Squeeze icing out of the cut corner, drizzling evenly over the top of the bars. Sprinkle chopped pecans over the bars.
9. For best results, let icing set for 1 hour or more. Store bars in an airtight container.

PER SERVING

Calories: 143| protein: 12g| carbs: 12g|fat: 6g

Chewy Banana Bites

Prep time: 10 minutes | Cook time: 15 minutes | Makes 12 bites

- ¼ cup whole unsalted almonds
- 2 large ripe bananas
- 1 cup plus 2 tablespoons rolled oats
- 4 teaspoons hemp hearts
- 2 tablespoons ground flaxseed
- 1 tablespoon vanilla extract
- 2 teaspoons ground cinnamon
- ⅛ teaspoon sea salt
- 2½ tablespoons 70% dark chocolate chips

1. Preheat the oven to 350°F. Line a baking sheet with parchment paper.
2. Put the almonds in a small zip-top plastic bag, seal, and crush them using a rolling pin.
3. In a large bowl, mash the bananas with a fork. Add the oats, hemp hearts, flaxseed, almonds, vanilla, cinnamon, and salt and mix well. Add the chocolate chips and mix until well combined.
4. Using your hands, form the mixture into 12 equal balls and place them on the prepared baking sheet. Using a spoon, gently press down on each ball to flatten the tops.
5. Bake for 15 minutes, or until slightly golden. Let the bites cool on a wire rack for 10 minutes before serving.
6. Store any leftover bites in an airtight container for up to 3 days.

PER SERVING (1 BITE)

Calories: 95| Fat: 4g| Total Carbohydrates: 13g| Net Carbs: 10g| Fiber: 3g| Protein: 3g| Sodium: 21mg

No-Bake Chocolate Protein Bars with Quinoa

Prep time: 25 minutes, plus time to chill | Cook time: 25 minutes | Serves 8

- 1/3 cup dry quinoa, rinsed
- 2/3 cup water
- 16 whole dates, pitted
- 1/2 cup raw almonds
- 1/2 cup almond butter, preferably crunchy
- 1/2 cup chocolate protein powder
- 1 tablespoon honey (optional)

1. Add quinoa and water to a medium pot; bring to a boil over medium heat. Cover with a lid, reducing heat to low so mixture is at a simmer. Let cook for 15 minutes before removing from the heat. Cool quinoa and refrigerate it a minimum of 2 hours or even overnight.
2. Add dates into the bowl of a food processor, pulsing to turn it into a paste. Transfer the date paste to a small bowl.
3. Next, add raw almonds into the food processor, pulsing until they break into small pieces but before they turn into flour. Return dates to the food processor bowl, along with reserved quinoa, almond butter, protein powder, and (optional) honey. Blend until ingredients are well combined.
4. Divide mixture into 8 parts and form each one into a bar shape. Refrigerate for 1 to 2 hours until hardened and store in an airtight container.

PER SERVING

Calories: 331| protein: 11g| carbs: 49g|fat: 13g

Savory Rosemary Almond Bars

Prep time 10 minutes | Cook time 35 minutes | Serves 8

- 2 cups whole almonds, finely chopped
- 2 tbsp coconut flour
- 1/2 cup almond flour
- 2 tbsp finely chopped fresh rosemary
- 1 tsp garlic powder
- 1 tsp onion flakes
- 1/2 cup liquid egg whites
- 3 tbsp coconut oil

1. Preheat the oven to 300°F (149°C). Line an 8 x 8in (20 x 20cm) baking dish with aluminum foil.
2. In a large bowl, combine the almonds, coconut flour, almond flour, rosemary, garlic powder, onion flakes, and salt. Mix well.
3. Add the egg whites and coconut oil. Using clean hands, mix the ingredients until they form a rough dough. Press the dough into the baking dish, ensuring the thickness is uniform throughout.
4. Bake for 30 minutes, or until the bars are lightly browned around the edges. Slice into 8 equal-sized bars.

PER SERVING

Calories: 269|fat:22.3g|carbs: 7.4g| protein: 14g

Maple-Walnut Protein Muffins

Prep time: 5 minutes | Cook time: 25 minutes, plus time to cool | Serves 12

- 3 egg whites or 1/2 cup liquid egg white substitute
- 3 tablespoons unsalted butter, softened
- 1/4 cup maple syrup
- 1/2 cup 2% milk
- 1/2 cup whole-wheat flour
- 1/4 cup wheat germ
- 1/4 cup oat bran
- 6 scoops chocolate protein powder
- 2 teaspoons baking powder
- 1 teaspoon baking soda
- 1/2 cup chopped walnuts

1. Preheat the oven to 350 degrees F. Line a standard 12-cup muffin pan with paper liners or lightly coat cups with cooking spray.
2. In a medium bowl, add egg whites, butter, maple syrup, and milk. Use a fork to mix well.
3. In a large bowl, add flour, wheat germ, oat bran, protein powder, baking powder, and baking soda. Combine with a spatula.
4. Using the spatula, add wet ingredients to the dry ingredients, stirring only until the dry ingredients are moistened. When there's just a trace of visible flour, gently fold in the nuts.
5. Divide batter among 12 prepared muffin cups, filling each cup three-fourths of the way full.
6. Bake until toasty brown on top and a toothpick inserted into the middle of a muffin comes out clean, about 20 to 25 minutes.
7. Let muffins cool for a few minutes before removing from the pan. Allow to fully cool before serving. Store remaining muffins in an airtight container.

PER SERVING

Calories: 176| protein: 15g| carbs: 15g|fat: 7g

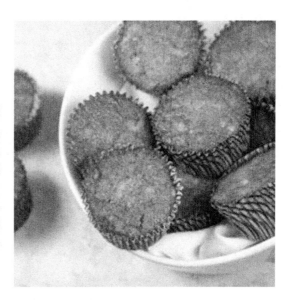

No-Bake Almond and Oats Bars

Prep time 40 minutes | Cook time 5 minutes| Serves 12

- 2 cups quick oats
- 3 scoops whey protein powder
- ½ cup creamy almond butter
- ⅔ cup almond milk
- 1 tsp vanilla extract
- 2 tbsp powdered stevia

1. In a large bowl, combine the oats, protein powder, almond butter, almond milk, vanilla extract, and stevia. Mix well until the ingredients form a dough.
2. Press the dough into a 9 x 13in (23 x 33cm) baking pan. Place the pan in the refrigerator for 30 minutes to harden the bars.
3. Cut into 8 equal-sized bars, and individually wrap in parchment paper. Seal the wrapped bars in a plastic storage bag.

PER SERVING

Calories:215 |fat:10g|carbs: 17.3g| protein: 14.3g

Pumpkin and Oat Bars

Prep time 10 minutes | Cook time 25 minutes| Serves 6

- 1 cup oat flour
- ½ cup vanilla whey protein powder
- 1 tsp baking powder
- ½ tsp salt
- 2 tsp ground cinnamon
- ½ tsp allspice
- ½ tsp ground ginger
- ⅓ cup powdered stevia
- ⅓ cup liquid egg whites
- 1 cup canned pumpkin purée (not pumpkin pie mix)
- 1 tsp vanilla extract

1. Preheat the oven to 350°F (177°C). Spray an 8 x 8in (20 x 20cm) baking pan with non-stick cooking spray.
2. In a large bowl, combine the oat flour, protein powder, baking powder, salt, cinnamon, allspice, ginger, and stevia. Mix well.
3. In a separate large bowl, combine the egg whites, pumpkin purée, and vanilla extract. Mix well.
4. Make the batter by adding the wet ingredients to the dry ingredients. Mix well to combine.
5. Pour the batter into the baking pan. Bake for 20 to 25 minutes, or until a toothpick inserted in the middle comes out clean. Slice into 6 equal-sized bars.

PER SERVING

Calories:153 |fat:0.5g|carbs: 24.7g| protein: 11.9g

No-Bake Matcha Green Tea Fudge Bars

Prep time: 10 minutes, overnight refrigeration | Cook time: 15 minutes| Serves 10

- 1/2 cup oat flour
- 1/3 cup almond butter
- 1 cup plus 2 tablespoons unsweetened almond milk
- 1 teaspoon granulated sugar
- Zest of 1 lemon
- 2 ounces dark chocolate, finely chopped

1. Prepare an 8-inch by 8-inch baking pan by lining it with parchment paper, using 2 sheets placed in opposite directions.
2. In a small bowl, add protein powder, matcha, and oat flour. Use a fork to thoroughly combine; reserve.
3. In the bowl of a stand mixer, add almond butter, almond milk, Stevia, and lemon zest. Mix on low to combine (or alternatively mix by hand with a spatula). Slowly add the protein powder mixture, stirring to combine.
4. Transfer matcha fudge to the prepared pan, using a spatula to evenly spread the mixture. Cover with plastic wrap and place in the fridge overnight.
5. Lift the parchment paper from the pan and place onto a cutting board. Slice fudge into 10 pieces.
6. Using either a microwave or double boiler on the stove, gently stir the chocolate until melted. Drizzle melted chocolate over the bars.
7. Store bars in an airtight container.

PER SERVING

Calories: 194| protein: 21g| carbs: 12g|fat: 7g

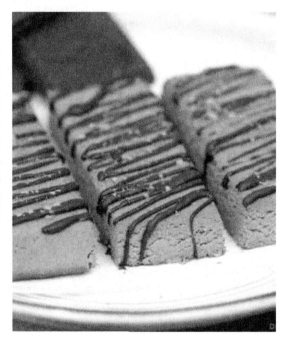

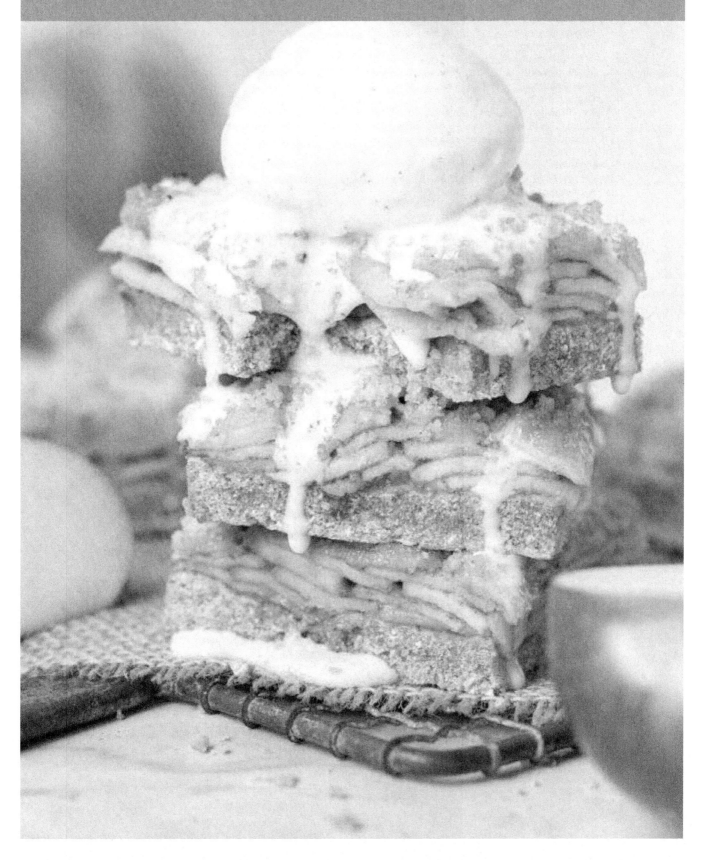

Drizzled Chocolate and Strawberries

Prep time: 5 minutes | Cook time: 1 minute | Serves 4

- 4 cups whole strawberries, rinsed and dried
- 2 ounces dark chocolate, broken into pieces

1. Line a baking sheet with parchment paper.
2. Put the strawberries on the prepared baking sheet.
3. In a microwave-safe bowl, melt the dark chocolate in 25-second intervals, stirring between each one, until smooth.
4. Using a spoon, quickly drizzle the chocolate over the strawberries. Refrigerate them for at least 30 minutes. Serve immediately or put them in an airtight container and refrigerate for up to 2 days.

PER SERVING

Calories: 131 | Fat: 6 g | Protein: 2 g | Sodium: 4 mg | Fiber: 4 g | Carbohydrates: 18 g | Sugar: 4 g

Salted Caramel Cashew Bites

Prep time: 10 minutes | Cook time: 0 minute | Serves 7

- 1 cup pitted dates
- 2 teaspoons vanilla extract
- 1 tablespoon water
- ⅓ cup unsalted cashews
- ¼ cup raisins
- ⅛ cup peanuts

1. In a medium bowl, soak the dates in hot water for 10 minutes.
2. In a food processor, combine the dates, vanilla, and 1 tablespoon of water and process until it forms a paste. You may need to stop and scrape down the sides.
3. Add the cashews, raisins, and peanuts and continue to pulse until blended. Using your hands, form the mixture into 7 balls and put them on a plate. Refrigerate for at least 20 minutes before serving.
4. Store them in an airtight container in the refrigerator for up to 3 days.

PER SERVING

Calories: 166 | Fat: 4 g | Protein: 2 g | Sodium: 3 mg | Fiber: 2 g | Carbohydrates: 2 g | Sugar: 4 g

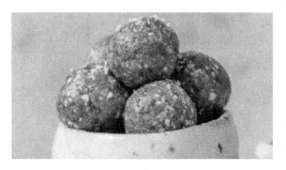

Cranberry Chocolate Cookies with Oats

Prep time: 10 minutes | Cook time: 20 minutes | Serves 12

- 1¼ cups all-purpose flour
- 1 cup rolled oats
- ¼ cup packed brown sugar
- ¼ cup salted pistachios
- ¼ cup dried cranberries
- 2 tablespoons dark chocolate chips
- 1 teaspoon baking powder
- ⅛ teaspoon sea salt
- 2 large eggs, beaten
- ¼ cup coconut oil, melted
- 1 teaspoon vanilla extract

1. Preheat the oven to 350°F (180°C). Line a baking sheet with parchment paper.
2. In a large bowl, mix the flour, oats, brown sugar, pistachios, cranberries, chocolate chips, baking powder, and salt.
3. In another bowl, mix the eggs, coconut oil, and vanilla. Pour the wet ingredients into the dry ingredients and mix until it forms a stiff dough. Using your hands, roll the mixture into 12 balls and put them on the prepared baking sheet. Using a spoon, flatten out the tops.
4. Bake for 18 to 20 minutes, or until lightly golden brown. Let cool on the baking sheet for 2 minutes before transferring them to a wire rack to cool completely. Store in an airtight container.

PER SERVING

Calories: 174| Fat: 7 g | Protein: 4 g | Sodium: 49 mg | Fiber: 2 g | Carbohydrates: 24 g | Sugar: 2 g

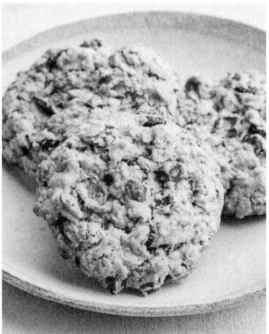

Chocolate Chips with Black Bean Brownie

Prep time: 10 minutes | Cook time: 25 minutes | Serves 8

- Nonstick cooking spray
- 1 (15-ounce) can black beans, drained and rinsed
- ½ cup rolled oats
- ⅓ cup maple syrup
- ¼ cup olive oil
- ¼ cup creamy 100% all-natural peanut butter
- 2 tablespoons unsweetened cocoa powder
- ½ tablespoon vanilla extract
- ½ teaspoon baking powder
- ½ cup dark chocolate chips
- ¼ cup chopped walnuts

1. Preheat the oven to 350°F. Lightly spray a 12-cup muffin tin with nonstick cooking spray. Set aside.
2. In a food processor, combine the black beans, oats, maple syrup, olive oil, peanut butter, cocoa powder, vanilla, and baking powder and pulse until well combined.
3. Add the chocolate chips and pulse until combined. Transfer the brownie batter to a large bowl and fold in the walnuts. Divide the batter equally between the muffin cups.
4. Bake for 20 to 25 minutes, or until cooked. Let cool for 10 minutes before serving.
5. Refrigerate the brownies in an airtight container for up to 4 days.

PER SERVING

Calories: 303 | Fat: 18 g | Protein: 8 g | Sodium: 6 mg | Fiber: 6 g | Carbohydrates: 29 g | Sugar: 3 g

Chocolate-Chia Mousse

Prep time: 10 minutes, plus 5 minutes to soak | Cook time: 45 minutes | Serves 8

- 2 tablespoons chia seeds
- ½ cup water
- 1 avocado
- 6 tablespoons unsweetened cocoa powder
- 1 teaspoon vanilla extract
- 6 egg whites
- ¼ teaspoon cream of tartar
- 1 cup granulated stevia, plus more for serving
- Fresh fruit, for serving (optional)
- Ground cinnamon, for serving (optional)

1. Preheat the oven to 350°F.
2. In a small bowl, soak the chia seeds in the water for about 5 minutes, until they form a gel.
3. In a food processor or blender, blend the chia gel, avocado, cocoa powder, and vanilla until smooth.
4. In a large bowl, whip the egg whites and cream of tartar until stiff peaks form. Gradually add the stevia and the chia–cocoa powder mixture.
5. Pour into 8 ramekins or a baking-cup-lined muffin tin. Place in a water bath (a larger pan filled with

water), and bake for 45 minutes.
6. The center will still be gooey. Transfer to the refrigerator for about 30 minutes to chill completely.
7. To serve, top with some fresh fruit or sprinkle with cinnamon and a little more stevia (remember to add calories from the fruit to the total).

PER SERVING

Calories: 70 |carbs: 5.1g|fat: 4.4g|protein 4.5g

Sugar, Gluten-Free Peanut Butter Cookies

Prep time: 10 minutes| Cook time: 10 minutes| Makes 16 cookies

- 1 egg white
- 1 tablespoon vanilla extract
- 1 tablespoon milled flaxseed
- 1 cup natural creamy peanut butter
- 1 cup granulated stevia

1. Preheat the oven to 350°F.
2. Line a cookie sheet with parchment paper or a silicone baking sheet.
3. In a small bowl, mix the egg white, vanilla, and flaxseed. Set aside to rest.
4. If any oil has separated from the peanut butter, mix together until smooth. In a large bowl, mix the peanut butter and stevia. Add the egg white mixture, and mix until smooth with no visible stevia granules.
5. Scoop out about 1 tablespoon of dough, and roll it into a ball; you should have about 16 even balls. Place the balls on the prepared sheet. Using a fork, make a crosshatch by gently pressing down in one direction, then again in another, making the crisscross pattern.
6. Bake for 8 to 12 minutes. Less time will give a softer cookie, more time will give a crispier cookie.
7. Cool for a few minutes before removing the cookies from the baking sheet and serving.

PER SERVING

Calories: 98 |carbs: 3.6g|fat:8g|protein :4.3g

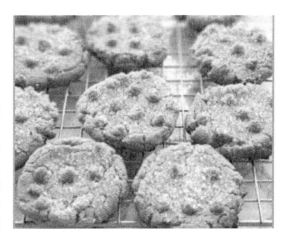

Perfect Pumpkin Pie

Prep time: 20 minutes| Cook time: 35 minutes | Serves 8

FOR THE CRUST

- 2 tablespoons psyllium husk
- ⅛ teaspoon xanthan gum
- ⅓ cup hot water
- 1¼ cups almond flour
- ½ cup unsalted raw almonds
- ½ cup corn starch
- ⅛ teaspoon salt
- ½ teaspoon baking soda
- 3 to 4 tablespoons water, if needed
- coconut oil, for greasing

FOR THE FILLING

- 1 (15-ounce) can 100% pure pumpkin
- ½ cup nonfat Greek yogurt
- 1 cup fat-free cottage cheese
- 1 cup (from 8 to 12 eggs) egg whites
- 3 teaspoons ground cinnamon
- 1 teaspoon ground allspice
- 1 teaspoon ground ginger
- 1 teaspoon ground nutmeg
- ½ teaspoon ground cloves
- ½ teaspoon salt
- 1 cup granulated stevia

TO MAKE THE CRUST

1. In a small bowl, mix the psyllium husk, xanthan gum, and hot water. Allow the mixture to sit and thicken for 5 minutes.
2. Meanwhile, in a blender or food processor, process the almond flour, almonds, corn starch, salt, and baking soda, stopping to stir and scrape down the sides as needed, until a fine flour forms.
3. Add the psyllium husk mixture to the food processor, and process. If the dough is still crumbly, add 1 tablespoon of water at a time, blending between additions, until the dough clumps together.
4. Place the dough on a piece of parchment paper or a silicone baking sheet, and roll into a 10-inch circle.
5. Place the dough in a lightly greased 9-inch pie tin using this easy trick with 2 pie tins: First, place 1 pie tin upside down on your work surface. Pick up the parchment paper with the dough, and drape it dough-side-down onto the overturned pie tin. Peel off the parchment paper, and place the second pie tin over the dough. Flip the whole thing over, and remove the inner pie tin. This may seem like extra work, but it does a great job of preventing rips or tears in the dough.

TO MAKE THE FILLING

6. In a blender or food processor, blend the pumpkin, yogurt, cottage cheese, egg whites, cinnamon, allspice, ginger, nutmeg, cloves, salt, and stevia on high for 2 to 3 minutes, until smooth. Pour the mixture over the crust.

7. Bake for 25 to 35 minutes, until small cracks start to form on the filling. If you gently shake the pie, the filling will still wiggle.
8. Remove the pie from the oven, and allow it to cool completely, about 30 minutes.
9. Cut into eight even slices and serve.

Per Serving
Calories: 215|carbs: 18g|fat: 10.7g|protein :12.9g

Raspberry Sorbet

Prep time: 3 minutes| Serves 1

- 1 cup frozen raspberries
- ½ cup sugar-free vanilla almond milk
- ¼ cup granulated stevia

1. In a food processor or blender, blend the raspberries, almond milk, and stevia until a thick, smooth texture is formed. You will have to shake or stir the ingredients a few times. Avoid the urge to add extra almond milk. It will make the sorbet runny.
2. Spoon into a serving bowl and enjoy.

PER SERVING

Calories: 85 |carbs:17g|fat: 2g|protein 2g

Peach Cobbler

Prep time: 15 minutes | Cook time: 35 minutes, plus 20 minutes resting | Serves 6

- 3 tablespoons blueberries, raspberries, strawberries, or mixed-fruit preserves
- 1 (15-ounce) can diced peaches in water or 100% juice, drained
- 1/2 cup 2% cottage cheese
- 1/2 cup water
- 2 scoops vanilla protein powder
- 1/4 cup all-purpose flour
- 1/3 cup Truvia
- 1/2 cup quick-cooking oats
- 1 tablespoon honey

1. Preheat the oven to 350 degrees F. Coat an 8-inch square baking dish with cooking spray.
2. Add the fruit preserves into the prepared dish and use a spatula to spread it evenly. Top with a layer of peaches and set aside.
3. In a medium bowl, add cottage cheese, water, protein powder, flour, and Truvia. Mix well and pour over the peaches.
4. In a small bowl, mix oats and honey. Spoon over the top of cobbler.
5. Bake until golden, around 30 minutes. Let sit for at least 20 minutes before serving.

PER SERVING

Calories:161 | protein: 12g| carbs: 28g|fat: 1g

Key Lime Pie

Prep time: 15 minutes, plus 4 to 6 hours to chill | Cook time: 55 minutes| Serves 6

- 3/4 cup honey graham cracker crumbs (about 4 sheets of crackers)
- 1/2 cup applesauce
- 1 cup quick-cooking oats
- 1 teaspoon ground cinnamon
- 3 large egg yolks
- 1 (14-ounce) can condensed milk
- ? cup key lime juice
- 2 cups frozen whipped topping, thawed in fridge for 4 to 5 hours

1. Preheat the oven to 350 degrees F.
2. In a large bowl, add graham cracker crumbs, applesauce, oats, and cinnamon. Mix well. Remove 1 tablespoon of the mixture and reserve in the refrigerator for later use.
3. Spread the graham cracker mixture into a 9-inch pie plate. Lightly press it along the bottom and sides to form the crust. Bake until edges are golden, about 15 minutes. When crust is done, reduce the oven temperature to 250 degrees F.
4. In a medium bowl, whisk egg yolks, condensed milk, and lime juice until smooth. Pour the lime juice mixture into the prepared crust. Bake until the filling is firm, about 40 minutes.
5. Remove the pie from the oven and cool completely. Refrigerate for 4 to 6 hours or until fully chilled. Top with a 2-inch layer of the whipped topping, sprinkle with reserved crumb mixture, and serve.

PER SERVING

Calories:475 | protein: 11g| carbs: 74g|fat: 16g

Sweet Potato Casserole

Prep time: 15 minutes | Cook time: 35 minutes| Serves 4

- 3 cups mashed sweet potatoes
- 1/3 cup skim milk
- 1 tablespoon melted unsalted butter
- 1 teaspoon vanilla extract
- 1/2 teaspoon salt
- 2 egg whites or 6 tablespoons liquid egg white substitute
- 1/4 cup packed brown sugar
- 1/4 cup all-purpose flour
- 1 tablespoon olive oil

1. Preheat the oven to 350 degrees F. Coat a 7-inch by 11-inch baking dish with cooking spray and set aside.
2. In a large bowl, add mashed sweet potatoes, milk, butter, vanilla, salt, and egg whites. Mix well and spread evenly into the prepared baking dish.
3. In a small bowl, add brown sugar and flour. Slowly drizzle in olive oil and stir until the mixture has the consistency of coarse crumbs.

4. Sprinkle the crumb mixture over sweet potatoes and bake for 30 minutes. Serve.

PER SERVING

Calories: 243| protein: 5g| carbs: 41g|fat: 7g

Maple-Raisin Bread Pudding

Prep time: 25 minutes, plus time to chill | Cook time: 55 minutes| Serves 4

- 2 cups 1/2-inch cubes French bread
- 1 cup skim milk
- 2 large eggs
- 2 1/2 teaspoons vanilla extract
- 4 tablespoons pure maple syrup, divided
- 1/3 cup raisins

1. Preheat the oven to 350 degrees F. Spread bread pieces onto a baking sheet, ensuring pieces don't touch. Toast in the oven, stirring after a couple minutes. Bake until golden, about 5 minutes, and then let cool.
2. In a large bowl, whisk together milk, eggs, vanilla, and 3 tablespoons maple syrup. Use a spatula to stir in raisins and gently fold in toasted bread. Cover and refrigerate for at least 30 minutes and up to 4 hours.
3. Preheat the oven to 325 degrees F. Coat 4 small ramekins with cooking spray and divide the mixture between them. Evenly space the ramekins in an 8-inch by 8-inch square baking pan and fill the pan with 1 inch of hot water.
4. Bake bread pudding until set, about 45 to 50 minutes. Drizzle the remaining 1 tablespoon maple syrup over the top and serve.

PER SERVING

Calories:277 | protein: 10g| carbs: 50g|fat: 3g

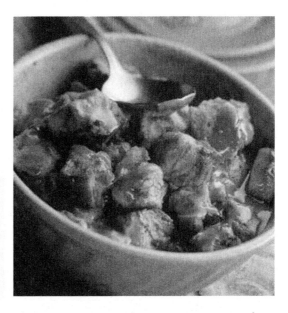

Mini Cheesecakes

Prep time: 35 minutes | Cook time: 15 minutes| Serves 6 (2 cheesecakes per serving)

- 1 (12-ounce) package vanilla wafers
- 2 (8-ounce) packages reduced-fat cream cheese
- 1/3 cup plus 1 tablespoon Truvia
- 2 large eggs
- 1 teaspoon vanilla extract

1. Preheat the oven to 350 degrees F. Line the cups of a standard 12-cup muffin pan with paper liners.
2. Make wafers into fine crumbs by pulsing in a food processor or adding into a large Ziploc bag, sealing tightly, and crushing with a rolling pin. Spoon 2 tablespoons into each muffin liner.
3. In a large bowl, add cream cheese, Truvia, eggs, and vanilla. Using a handheld mixer, blend until light and fluffy.
4. Fill each muffin liner almost to the top with the cream cheese mixture.
5. 5 Bake until set, around 15 minutes. Remove from the oven and let cool before serving.

PER SERVING

Calories:567 | protein: 9g| carbs: 79g|fat: 24g

Triple Berry Crisp

Prep time: 25 minutes | Cook time: 45 minutes| Serves 6

- 3/4 cup blackberries
- 3/4 cup raspberries
- 3/4 cup blueberries
- 1 tablespoon granulated sugar
- 3/4 cup Truvia
- 1 cup whole-wheat flour
- 1 cup rolled oats
- 1/2 teaspoon ground cinnamon
- 1/4 teaspoon ground nutmeg
- 1/2 cup (1 stick) cold butter, cubed

1. Preheat oven to 350 degrees F. Coat a 9-inch by 13-inch pan with cooking spray.
2. In a large bowl, gently toss together blackberries, raspberries, and blueberries with 1 tablespoon sugar.
3. In another large bowl, combine Truvia with flour, oats, cinnamon, and nutmeg. Add cubed butter, using a fork to combine butter into mixture until crumbly.
4. Press half the oat mixture into the bottom of the prepared pan. Cover with berries and sprinkle remaining oat mixture on top.
5. Bake until fruit is bubbling and topping is golden brown, about 30 to 40 minutes.

PER SERVING

Calories: 524| protein: 6g| carbs: 92g|fat: 17g

Greek Yogurt "Cheesecake" with Chocolate Protein Crumb Crust

Prep time: 10 minutes| Cook time: 50 minutes | Serves 9

FOR THE CRUST

- ¼ cup almond flour
- ½ cup chocolate whey protein isolate
- ¼ cup unsweetened cocoa powder
- 3 tablespoons milled flaxseed
- ¼ cup granulated stevia or Splenda
- 3 tablespoons coconut oil, melted

FOR THE FILLING

- 2 eggs
- 2 cups nonfat Greek yogurt
- 1 teaspoon vanilla
- ½ cup granulated stevia
- 1 tablespoon gluten-free all-purpose baking mix
- Sugar-free jelly, for serving (optional)

1. Preheat the oven to 300°F.

TO MAKE THE CRUST

2. In a medium bowl, mix the almond flour, whey protein, cocoa powder, flaxseed, and stevia. Gradually add the melted coconut oil, and mix until large crumbs form.
3. Transfer to an ungreased 8-by- 8-inch pan, spreading over the bottom and pressing the crumb mixture firmly down to form an even crust.

TO MAKE THE FILLING

4. In a medium bowl, beat the eggs. Add the yogurt, and mix until smooth. Add the vanilla, and then gradually stir in the stevia and baking mix. Pour the mixture into the crust.
5. Bake for 45 to 50 minutes, until the center is firm.
6. Allow to cool completely, about 30 minutes.
7. Cut into nine even slices and serve plain or with a sugar-free jelly.

PER SERVING

Calories: 145 |carbs: 5.9g|fat: 8.8g|protein :13.2g

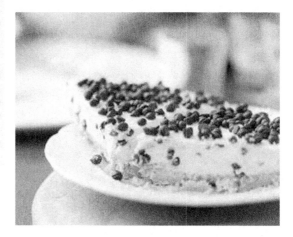

Bananas Foster

Prep time: 5 minutes | Cook time: 15 minutes | Serves 2

- 1/4 cup vegetable oil
- 1/3 cup dark brown sugar, unpacked
- 1 tablespoon bourbon vanilla extract
- 1/2 teaspoon ground cinnamon
- 2 ripe bananas, peeled and sliced lengthwise and then crosswise
- 1/4 cup coarsely chopped macadamia nuts
- 1 cup low-fat vanilla frozen yogurt

1. Warm oil in a large skillet over medium heat. Stir in brown sugar, vanilla, and cinnamon.
2. When the sugar mixture begins to bubble, stir in bananas and nuts. Cook until bananas are hot, 1 to 2 minutes.
3. Remove bananas from the heat and serve over a small scoop of frozen yogurt.

PER SERVING

Calories: 693 | protein: 6g | carbs: 76g | fat: 44g

Homemade Cinnamon-Spiced Applesauce

Prep time: 5 minutes, plus time to chill | Cook time: 25 minutes | Serves 4

- 4 apples, peeled, cored, and chopped
- 1/2 cup water
- 1/4 cup Truvia
- 1/2 teaspoon ground cinnamon

1. In a medium pot, combine apples, water, Truvia, and cinnamon.
2. Cover with a lid and cook over medium heat until apples are soft and break down, about 15 to 20 minutes.
3. Allow to cool and then mash with a fork or potato masher. Refrigerate until chilled and serve.

PER SERVING

Calories: 96 | protein: 1g | carbs: 25g | fat: 0g

Flourless Chocolate Cake

Prep time: 15 minutes | Cook time: 35 minutes, plus 10 minutes to cool | Serves 4

- 1/3 cup unsalted butter, plus more for greasing
- 4 ounces 80% dark chocolate, finely chopped
- 1/2 cup Truvia
- 1/2 cup unsweetened cocoa powder
- 3 large eggs, beaten
- 1 teaspoon vanilla extract

1. Preheat the oven to 300 degrees F. Grease an 8-inch round cake pan with butter.
2. In a heatproof medium bowl, add chocolate and butter. Gently warm in the microwave until melted. Stir in Truvia, cocoa powder, eggs, and vanilla. Pour into prepared pan.
3. Bake for 30 minutes. Remove from the oven and let cool for 10 minutes.
4. Remove cake from the pan onto a wire rack and let cool completely. Serve and enjoy.

PER SERVING

Calories: 377 | protein: 9g | carbs: 14g | fat: 34g

Classic Tiramisu

Prep time: 25 minutes, plus time to chill | Cook time: 15 minutes | Serves 8

- 1 (8-ounce) container reduced-fat cream cheese, softened
- 1/2 (8-ounce) container mascarpone cheese
- 1/2 cup Truvia
- 1 tablespoon brewed espresso or Kahlúa (optional)
- 24 ladyfingers
- 1 cup espresso, brewed and cooled
- 1 tablespoon Kahlúa
- 1 tablespoon packed brown sugar
- 1 1/2 teaspoons unsweetened cocoa powder
- 1/2 ounce bittersweet chocolate, grated

1. To make the filling, add cream cheese and mascarpone into a large bowl and use a handheld mixer to beat at medium speed until smooth. Add Truvia and 1 tablespoon brewed espresso or Kahlúa, if desired, beating at medium speed until blended.
2. Cut ladyfingers in half lengthwise. Arrange 24 ladyfinger halves, cut-side up, in the bottom of an 8-inch square baking dish.
3. In a small bowl, mix 1 cup espresso, 1 tablespoon Kahlúa, and brown sugar. Pour half the mixture over the ladyfingers to soak them; then spread a layer of half the cream cheese filling on top.
4. Repeat procedure with remaining 24 ladyfinger halves, soaking with the remaining espresso mixture and then topping with remaining cream cheese filling.
5. In a small bowl, combine cocoa and grated chocolate; sprinkle evenly over top of filling.
6. Cover with plastic wrap and chill for 2 hours or overnight. Cut and serve.

PER SERVING

Calories: 227 | protein: 5g | carbs: 21g | fat: 13g

Appendix 1 Measurement Conversion Chart

Volume Equivalents (Dry)	
US STANDARD	METRIC (APPROXIMATE)
1/8 teaspoon	0.5 mL
1/4 teaspoon	1 mL
1/2 teaspoon	2 mL
3/4 teaspoon	4 mL
1 teaspoon	5 mL
1 tablespoon	15 mL
1/4 cup	59 mL
1/2 cup	118 mL
3/4 cup	177 mL
1 cup	235 mL
2 cups	475 mL
3 cups	700 mL
4 cups	1 L

Volume Equivalents (Liquid)		
US STANDARD	US STANDARD (OUNCES)	METRIC (APPROXIMATE)
2 tablespoons	1 fl.oz.	30 mL
1/4 cup	2 fl.oz.	60 mL
1/2 cup	4 fl.oz.	120 mL
1 cup	8 fl.oz.	240 mL
1 1/2 cup	12 fl.oz.	355 mL
2 cups or 1 pint	16 fl.oz.	475 mL
4 cups or 1 quart	32 fl.oz.	1 L
1 gallon	128 fl.oz.	4 L

Temperatures Equivalents	
FAHRENHEIT(F)	CELSIUS(C) APPROXIMATE)
225 °F	107 °C
250 °F	120 ° °C
275 °F	135 °C
300 °F	150 °C
325 °F	160 °C
350 °F	180 °C
375 °F	190 °C
400 °F	205 °C
425 °F	220 °C
450 °F	235 °C
475 °F	245 °C
500 °F	260 °C

Weight Equivalents	
US STANDARD	METRIC (APPROXIMATE)
1 ounce	28 g
2 ounces	57 g
5 ounces	142 g
10 ounces	284 g
15 ounces	425 g
16 ounces (1 pound)	455 g
1.5 pounds	680 g
2 pounds	907 g

Appendix 2 The Dirty Dozen and Clean Fifteen

The Environmental Working Group (EWG) is a nonprofit, nonpartisan organization dedicated to protecting human health and the environment Its mission is to empower people to live healthier lives in a healthier environment. This organization publishes an annual list of the twelve kinds of produce, in sequence, that have the highest amount of pesticide residue-the Dirty Dozen-as well as a list of the fifteen kinds ofproduce that have the least amount of pesticide residue-the Clean Fifteen.

THE DIRTY DOZEN	
The 2016 Dirty Dozen includes the following produce. These are considered among the year's most important produce to buy organic:	
Strawberries	Spinach
Apples	Tomatoes
Nectarines	Bell peppers
Peaches	Cherry tomatoes
Celery	Cucumbers
Grapes	Kale/collard greens
Cherries	Hot peppers
The Dirty Dozen list contains two additional itemskale/collard greens and hot peppers-because they tend to contain trace levels of highly hazardous pesticides.	

THE CLEAN FIFTEEN	
The least critical to buy organically are the Clean Fifteen list. The following are on the 2016 list:	
Avocados	Papayas
Corn	Kiw
Pineapples	Eggplant
Cabbage	Honeydew
Sweet peas	Grapefruit
Onions	Cantaloupe
Asparagus	Cauliflower
Mangos	
Some of the sweet corn sold in the United States are made from genetically engineered (GE) seedstock. Buy organic varieties of these crops to avoid GE produce.	

Appendix 3 Index

DINO C. WRIGHT

Printed in Great Britain
by Amazon

21450254R00072